ESSENTIAL OILS

Essential Oils Beginners Guide for Weight Loss and Stress Relief

(Simple Homemade Essential Oils Natural Remedies to Improve Your Health)

Matthew Powers

Published By Zoe Lawson

Matthew Powers

All Rights Reserved

Essential Oils: Essential Oils Beginners Guide for Weight Loss and Stress Relief (Simple Homemade Essential Oils Natural Remedies to Improve Your Health)

ISBN 978-1-77485-291-0

Legal & Disclaimer

The information contained in this book is not designed to replace or take the place of any form of medicine or professional medical advice. The information in this book has been provided for educational and entertainment purposes only.

The information contained in this book has been compiled from sources deemed reliable, and it is accurate to the best of the Author's knowledge; however, the Author cannot guarantee its accuracy and validity and cannot be held liable for any errors or omissions. Changes are periodically made to this book. You must consult your doctor or get professional medical advice before using any of the suggested remedies, techniques, or information in this book.

Upon using the information contained in this book, you agree to hold harmless the Author from and against any damages, costs, and expenses, including any legal fees potentially resulting from the application of any of the information provided by this guide. This disclaimer applies to any damages or injury caused by the use and application, whether directly or indirectly, of any advice or information presented, whether for breach of contract, tort, negligence, personal injury, criminal intent, or under any other cause of action.

You agree to accept all risks of using the information presented inside this book. You need to consult a professional medical practitioner in order to ensure you are both able and healthy enough to participate in this program.

TABLE OF CONTENTS

Introduction

The "Essential oils" book offers practical steps and tips for using essential oils for aromatherapy and beauty reasons. It is crucial that anyone starting out has an understanding of the different techniques and reasons for using these essential oils in order to make use of them in a proper manner. This book you'll learn:

1. Essential oils basics

2. The benefits of aromatherapy

3. The advantages of going organic

4. Oil pulling secrets

5. Coconut oil's numerous advantages

6. Herbal remedies that are fascinating and intriguing

7. A fresh approach to losing weight.

8. Blood sugar solutions

9. An anti aging miracle

10. Amazing cures for pets

Along with other details that will help you maximise the positive effects of your essential oil.

Chapter 1: Safety And Preparations

As the most concentrated form that the plants can produce, it is likely to be volatile however this is not the way that it can explode into your face.

Simple rules

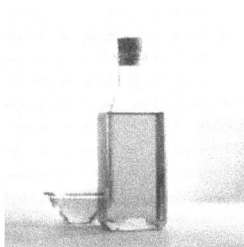

Always wear gloves while mixing essential oils and creating blends. This will ensure you do not suffer from contact dermatitis.

Make sure to keep vital oils from reach of your children. as well as pets.

Keep them in a cool and dark area. They'll evaporate even in the bottle when exposed to temperatures that are high.

NEVER use essential oils undiluted. There are websites which will inform you that it's okay to do this. It's not.

Do the Patch test

Every skin reacts differently to essential oils. Certain skin types are sensitive and develop blisters or a red rash. This is is known as contact dermatitis. Conducting a patch test will aid in determining whether you are able to apply the oil or not it. The neighborhood health store, or herbal shop will guide you on how to conduct an effective patch test.

Carrier oils

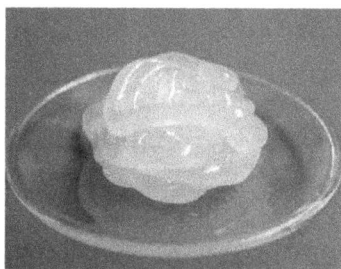

These are the oils you can use to dilute essential oils and create blends. There are a variety of carrier oils. However, I will only identify the most common here.

Sweet Almond oil

This is the most well-known base or carrier oil that is available. It's a light-weight oil, which means it doesn't require mixing the oil with any other and it's packed with proteins that are suitable for all types of skin.

Apricot Kernel Oil

It's a great alternative to the above for those who are intolerant to trees nuts. Although it's not as rich in the same proteins as Sweet Almond oil, it has minerals and vitamins that are beneficial for all skin types.

Cold-pressed Sesame oil

The base oil has to be combined with the other two mentioned above in a 10 percent solution. It has ingredients that can help fight inflammation caused by arthritis as well as Rheumatism, which causes joint pain.

How much do I use?

Everything must be accurately measured essential oils are no distinct from other essential oils. This list will help you determine the correct measurement of essential oils. When you're ready to strike out and create your own blends

One teaspoon Carrier, 2-5 drops Essential Oil (Essential Oil)

1 teaspoon of Carrier: 6- 15 drops EO

5ml of EO= 1 teaspoon

15ml of EO = 1 tablespoon

If you are looking to supplement essential oils with more than one carrier oil, here's the measurement scale you need:

20 drops EO = 1/5 TSP

40 drops EO = 2/5 TSP

60 drops EO = 3/5 TSP

There are between 50 and 75 drops the bottle of carrier which weighs 4 pounds.

Although it may appear that you're using lots of something, it could cost a lot according to the oil you use be aware that you'll be mixing various essential oils. Therefore, a small amount can go a long way. Also, you won't use essential oil preparations in large quantities.

tools of the Trade

Every new pastime requires the right equipment to succeed, and learning a new skill is the same. Here's a list of what you're likely to require to begin making the essential oil preparations.

Glass pot/Double boiler

Wooden or glass stirrers/spatulas

Glass funnel

Mesh filter

Dark glass containers with lids

Measurement of cups and spoons.

Mixing bowls

Epsom Salts

Sea Salt

Ground, steel cut oats

Borax

Glass is the preferred choice because of the petroleum nature of plastics and the capacity for liquids to remove the metal's properties. If you're using wooden spoons, use only to making mixtures and preparations. Be sure to avoid cross-contamination as far as you can.

Preparation

There's a lot of things to do, but I will just list the ones that are most beneficial to you.

Massage oils

These are the easiest of the three recipes.

They are created through the direct addition of essential oils to carriers oils.

They can be used in the form of massaging just a little portion of the mixture into the painful region.

Mineral Baths

They can ease discomfort and aches while enjoying the relaxation of soaking in a bath.

Pour 1/4 cup of the mixture into hot running water. A maximum of 1/2 cup is required.

These can be made from either salts or oatmeal in the case of hypertension.

Ointments

You can place them directly on the areas of pain.

This is a mix of non-petroleum jelly as well as essential oils

The oils will stay in the area for longer, allowing the healing process continue.

Salves

A salve is a heftier version of an oil.

It's also put in the area directly over your skin in order to speed the healing process.

It is produced by mixing beeswax and oils in a double-boiler and later adding Essential oils while it cools.

Chapter 2: Aromatherapy Secrets For Natural Beauty And Health

Aromatherapy is a popular method to help relax and put you at peace, but do you realize that aromatherapy can also be utilized as an organic beauty treatment? What about as a natural supplement to health? In this section, we'll look at the various essential oils as well as their impact upon our body.

Lemon essential oil. It's possible to think that the use of oil to combat oily skin might be strange, but that's precisely the purpose of this essential oil. It can help reduce the production of oil on your skin without drying it out , which is what most synthetic skin care products can do. Simply rub a couple of drops onto the areas of your skin that are problematic (make sure to dilute it!) and you're set to go.

Lavender essential oil. Do you want to find some nourishment and moisture on your skin? Lavender essential oil could be the ideal choice to accomplish this. It's a lot better than your typical lotion as it keeps your skin moisturized for hours. You don't need to apply any other lotion. It's also the most effective scar reduction products apply it to the affected area at least once each day and you'll notice a significant improvements in the appearance of your skin.

Peppermint essential oil. We know that it can help to calm our brains, but did you not know that it can have the similar impact to our stomachs. The addition of a drop of food grade essential oil of peppermint to tea could aid in digestion as inhaling its scent can calm an upset stomach. For those who are trying to lose weight, having a bit of it in your bag as an inhaler could reduce the desire to snack.

Rosemary Essential oil. Do you have dandruff problems? Don't fret! Take a few drops of it and gently rub the scalp with it; allow it to be within your hair for at most 30 minutes prior to washing it off with warm water. It is also possible to mix a bit of it in with your preferred shampoo. A few drops will suffice.

Chamomile essential oil. The tea-based version is known to cause sleepiness, so it's not surprise to know that the essential oils that are derived from it could perform the same function. Are you having trouble sleeping? Add the drops to your bath and then soak into it for at minimum 30 minutes. Not only will your tight muscles relax, but you'll also start getting sleepy after a few minutes. It's far superior to any sleep pill you can purchase.

Rose otto essential oil. PMS troubling you? Don't go for Tylenol right now. Give this oil a go and rub it into your neck and shoulders, it will help relieve the symptoms that accompany the pains that come with each month. It also smells wonderful!

Cedarwood essential oil. It is known to be extremely therapeutic and soothing for the body, this is a great oil to use on exhausted muscles and to help ease arthritis. If you are a regular exerciser, then you'll be aware of the pain that comes from muscle soreness when you massage your muscles using this can certainly ease the pain. Another use it's suitable for is to ease the symptoms associated with urinary and kidney tract infections. Add a few drops into a warm bath and let it soak for at least 30 minutes.

Jasmin essential oil. Are you feeling a bit down and tired? Apply just a few drops of the essential oil. It can help to clear your head and help you get into more tranquility. Inhaling the scent of jasmine can produce the same effect ideal for those who suffer from high levels of stress and are looking to unwind towards the close of their day. Jasmine can also boost the libido of females and males, so the use of it as an aromatherapy oil can be beneficial.

Geranium essential oil. To treat cellulite, this will be one of the most effective oils to apply. Apply a few drops of the oil and apply it to the affected area twice per every day. Within one week or so (depending on the degree that you have cellulite) you'll notice a noticeable improvement.

Tea tree essential oil. If you've used natural remedies for acne (or even bought ones) then you've known how effective the essential oil can be to tackling the issue. It has been scientifically proven to combat acne, without causing damage on the face. All you have just add some drops into your moisturizing cream or preferred carrier oil, and then apply it to problem areas.

Frankincense essential oil. Do you want to improve your immune system? This is the most essential oil for the job. It's an antiseptic and disinfectant that gets rid of the bacteria in the area you're in. It is also applied to injuries to help promote healing. It's also capable of protecting you from Tetanus.

Black pepper essential oil. It aids digestion, and at the exact helping to eliminate the toxins in your body. If you've felt gassy and bloated, this could be an option to eliminate these. It can also benefit people with arthritis or rheumatism, by getting rid of the root cause of the issue, such as the uric acid as well as other toxins that could cause the symptoms.

Cinnamon essential oil. Most often, it is used as a brain tonic it can be effective in treating respiratory disorders, issues that involve the circulation of blood, impurities and diabetes, and menstrual issues. It can also be utilized to alleviate bad breath!

Chapter 3: Essential Oil And Weight Loss

Essential oils can be very beneficial in helping you shed weight as they target the part of your brain that controls satisfaction and feeling along with the breaking down and elimination of undesirable fat and toxins from the body. Let's explore the different ways essential oils help you lose weight.

The use of essential oils in reducing appetite and achieving Satisfaction

The feeling of fullness generally controlled by a component of the hypothalamus located in the brain. Our nose and the olfactory nervous system is also linked to this area, and that our smell sense is tied to the hypothalamus within the brain. Aromatic oils emit scent-related molecules, which travel into in the nasal cavity and then the mucous membrane, and finally to the Olfactory nerve. These molecules are then absorbed into the limbic lobe of the brain, allowing the brain to react to the stimulus. The limbic lobe, which is the central nervous system's emotional center it relays information to the hypothalamus which can give you a feeling of being full.

The state of your mind can easily trigger the need to eat. Food chains and restaurants utilize essential oils to prepare of food, which can trigger cravings. You can also utilize the smell of food to help us and reduce our emotional reaction to food and our appetite. It is possible to use different essential oils to reduce appetite and help achieve satisfaction.

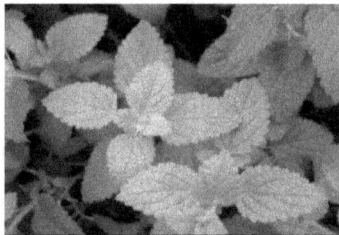

Peppermint

One of the most commonly utilized essential oils that aids in weight loss is peppermint. Studies have shown that peppermint has an influence in the hypothalamus. Inhaling the essential oil of peppermint prior to eating or placing some drops into the glass of water and drinking it before eating will provide you with the sensation of feeling full.

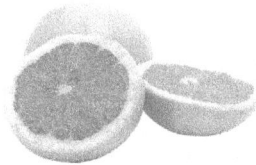

Grapefruit

Essential oils of grapefruit are helpful in cleansing the body of fluids and toxic substances. The scent reduces cravings for food and is therefore beneficial for weight loss. It is recommended to inhale grapefruit essential oil whenever cravings hit. It is also possible to put drops from the essential oil into the water in a glass to quell cravings.

Rosemary

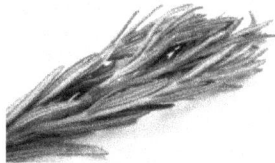

Rosemary is well-known for its effects on the mind and the memory. Additionally, it functions like an appetite suppressor since its hypothalamus is stimulated. In addition to enhancing appetite it also aids in detoxification.

This helps the body to eliminate excess fluids and toxic toxins. It also aids in the digestion of food. It is recommended to keep an oil bottle on hand and take a sniff at the oil when you feel hungry. Sniff three times through both nostrils.

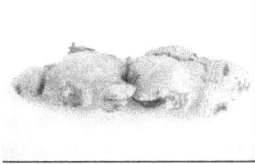

Ginger

Ginger can be used as an appetite suppressant. It can also aid in improving your digestion, and increases your energy levels as well. However, you must take care when using it as it can cause burning. Similar to as with any other essential oil that is that is used to suppress appetite, make sure you keep it in your hand and smell it whenever the urge to eat strikes.

Lime

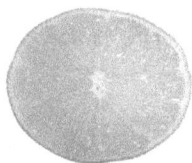

Essential oil of Lime is crucial in fighting cellulite because it's rich in vitamin C. The aroma of the oil is helpful in treating depression as well as encouraging positive thinking. This means that not only will it assist in eliminating cellulite but also helps to prevent the urge to eat a lot as it lifts your spirits.

Basil

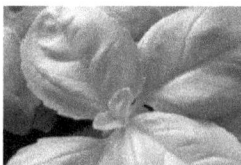

Basil is most effective as a fat-burner when combined with carrier oil. When you have the mix prepared, you can massage the oil all over your body. This will help to melt the fat in your body and will help you lose weight.

Thyme

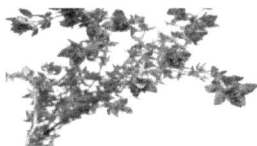

Thyme has numerous beneficial properties that make it a potent allies in healing. As a stimulant it helps to stimulate the digestive system, which in turn improves metabolism. This is extremely beneficial to people who are trying to lose weight.

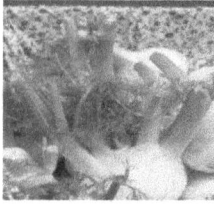

Fennel

Fennel is also known to stimulate the hypothalamus to create feelings of satiety. It means that after taking a breath you'll feel fuller and not crave food. Fennel can also help to boost the positive energy. This is particularly beneficial to those who gain weight through comfort food as an optimistic outlook can reduce your craving for comfort food. It is recommended to sniff the oil at least once throughout the day.

Once you start using essential oils to reduce your appetite, then you'll have to select at least three oils to use throughout the day. It is recommended that you carry them everywhere you go and to use often, since they have been proven to be beneficial with repeated usage. If you notice that you're in a mood to eat or getting hungry, or prior to eating your meal, open the bottle and take about three sniffs through each nostril. You should take as deep a breath as you can in each nostril while you close the other. After you've finished closing the bottle as soon as you can to prevent dispersing the scent. It is recommended to alternate the essential oils in order to keep from becoming accustomed to one particular oil in the sense that it ceases to have any effects. It is possible to inhale several times a day or add some drops of it into water and drink it based on the needs of your body.

Chapter 4: The Mother's Boob and Stomach Rub

This rub is perfect for moms who are pregnant. Since breasts and tummies grow during the course of pregnancy and breastfeeding this ointment can help to maintain the health on your skin. Cocoa butterand shea butter olive oil, vitamin E are all commonly utilized in a variety of skin ointments that are available for sale. They are all safe oils to use when pregnant or post-birth.

What you'll require:

8 oz glass container

White covers or any color you prefer

1 cup of cocoa butter

1 cup of shea butter

1/4 cup olive oil

1 TB of vitaminE

3 drops of oil from geranium

3 drops of lavender oil

Instructions:

Place your cocoa and butter in a double-burner on low heat , and allow the fats to melt. Remove the pan from the flame and place them in the dish of a tumbler. Cool, and then add Vitamin E, olive oil, and other oils. Keep it in the fridge for at least 60 hours or so until the mixture begins to firm up. After that, take it out from the fridge and mix the mixture in the blender until it forms the appearance of whipped cream. Scoop into your glass container. Securely seal and store in an area that is cool and dark. Massage the tummy and boobs every day whenever needed.

Lethargic Spray

I love this blend to aid me in sleeping. It's a soothing, calming spray that mixes certain oils with a certain type of magnesium. We are often deficient in the mineral due to the effects of our depleted soils and poor nutrition. Magnesium can also be calming It's an added dose of tranquil bliss!

The secret ingredient in this formula lies in the magnesium oil, which functions like a "transporter oil." This magnesium-rich transdermal source is less irritant to your body and is more gentle than that is taken orally.

You'll need:

2 ounce dim glass shower bottle

About 2 1 oz. of magnesium oil, an old mineral

20 drops of peace and calm (you could also try lavender, cedarwood, tangerine or roman chamomile, german or german.) oil

Instructions:

Fill your bottle with magnesium oil. Include your essential oils. Place the top on the splash bottle and shake thoroughly. Apply for 20 minutes prior to bed. Or, take a deep breath and open the bottle. into the scent as an aid to calming.

Bubble Baths

There is nothing that can rival the joy of a bath. I remember being surrounded by bubbles in my parents' bath, molding Santa Claus beards and making castles and towers out of bubbles. This is among my very favorite childhood memories.

Why am I not allowing my children to experience this?

A lot of bubble bath products available are today containing a number of horrendous substances... fragrances and parabens, some even formaldehyde.

But, will this inconvenience hinder an obstinate mother and her children's bath time? No, not in my house!

Create your own Bubble Bath

The best option is to create the bubble bath yourself! This is a top choice for DIYers or those who want to make sure your bubble bath is free of toxic chemicals or poisons.

The formulas listed here are three or two strategies to test.

Relaxing Salt Bubble Bath

The addition of magnesium-rich salt provides this bath a relaxing and revitalizing boost. It is a great way to soothe children and easing growing discomfort!

1/2 cup epsom salt or magnesium flakes

1/8 cup himalayan pink salt (not obligatory)

1 cup liquid castile soap

1 tbsp. vegetable glycerin

30-50 drops essential Oils

Mix all the ingredients together. Pour the mixture over running water, as you fill the bath.

Moisturizing Honey Bubble Bath

The almond oil and honey included in the recipe is great for moisturizing dry skin and for children suffering from eczema.

1 Cup sweet almond oil

1/2 cup honey

3/4 cup liquid castile soap

30-50 drops of essential oils (Lavender is a good choice)

Combine all the ingredients. Sprinkle the mixture on top of running water as you fill the bathtub.

Super Bubble Bath

The egg white used in this recipe aids in helping the bubbles retain their shape longer.

1 cup liquid castile cleaning soap

1 egg white

30-50 drops essential oils

Mix all the ingredients together. Pour the mixture over running water before adding the water to your bath. To boost the amount of foam Add a small amount of water and mix it with the aid of a hand mixer to produce additional foam prior to filling the bath.

You could include 1 cup of liquid to extend the recipe to extend the time it takes to cook. It won't be as bubbly, but it will cost less money.

We have a reason why we don't allow our children to take baths

Bathing in bubbles is a great thing but you must limit them to every week for your family.

The skin is home to beneficial bacteria that shouldn't get removed too often. This is why skin-to-skin contact is crucial for newborns who are creating their microbiome.

The "hygiene theory" suggests that the insufficient exposure to pathogens and microorganisms during the first year of life could cause harm to the development of the immune system. The results of research have shown that excessive bathing could result in eczema and asthma bronchial, leukaemia as well as diabetes.

The regular oil (sebum) in our pores could cause dry skin, or trigger the skin to go into sebum overdrive , which can lead in oily, greasy skin.

Additionally, the natural oils that we apply to our skin aid in the absorbance from Vitamin D that is derived from sunlight. Your skin could take up for up to 48 hours in order to fully absorb vitamin D through your skin, and washing it too often could negatively impact your Vitamin D levels.

There's a bit of a downer about bubble baths, isn't it? Butin moderation bubble baths can be very healthy and fun.

Mommy enjoys a nice bubble bath as well!

You're never older than your own private bubble bath! I prefer adding the occasional drop in Lavender, Chamomile Peace & Calming or Stress Away essential oils to the bath I take to provide an additional sense of relaxation.

What do you think?

Do your kids take bubble baths? What bubble bath do make use of?

Chapter 5: 10 Essential Oils You Can Trust to help burn fat, boost metabolism and Stress Relieve Stress

Essential oils have proven to be highly efficient in losing weight and controlling it. They are especially effective when combined with a well-balanced diet and lifestyle. Essential oils are always in handy because they help melt away fat and also assist the body in removing toxic substances. Essential oils are natural and don't cause any side consequences like other weight loss products.

Healthy weight management requires the correct techniques and oils have been proven over time to be effective. To work to help you lose weight , essential oils aid in reducing appetite, increasing metabolism, improving digestion blood sugar control, and also helping to regulate your mood. Therefore, it is recommended to lose weight, you mix essential oils along with a balanced diet and regular exercises.

Stress is a state which everyone fears because it could completely change the way you live and can be the source of many diseases e.g. depression, heart disease. Stress is caused by the way that the body responds issues and when the stress persists, it could seriously harm your health. Essential oils are being promoted as a fantastic method to combat stress because they have certain substances that can help to relax and stimulate.

Essential oils can work in a different way for each person based on what they require to enable their equilibrium and balance to return. Patients who are stressed will receive calm, whereas a bored one will experience a regaining. It's helpful to know that when you are making application of essential oils, they are extremely convenient, fast and simple to apply. If you're able to reduce stress, you can easily keep your body in good shape and well-maintained.

Metabolism is the term used to describe all the chemical reactions occurring in an organism in which complicated molecules break down down to create energy. It also can be utilized to create complicated body molecules. It's basically the process of turning food into energy. There aren't any specific oils that can be utilized to help burn fat, however certain essential oils that increase your metabolism and help you shed weight and lose fat.

The essential 10 oils that aid in burning fat, stress relief , and metabolism are listed below The essential oils listed below are:

Grapefruit essential oil.

Lemon essential oil.

Bergamot essential oil.

Lavender essential oil.

Peppermint essential oil.

Cypress essential oil.

Basil essential oil.

Cinnamon essential oil.

Oregano essential oil.

Rosemary essential oil.

Grapefruit essential oil

It is generally made by pressing the rind of the fruit the fruit. It has a fresh crisp and fresh aroma. Its properties make it possible to be extremely beneficial for anyone trying to reduce their body weight. The scent of grapefruit boosts stamina and energy levels, increasing your levels of energy in the process. Essential oils of grapefruit are recognized as being extremely effective in regulating metabolism, as it assists in cleaning the system. The scent provides people with spiritual and emotional support , which is why it's so effective for relieving stress. It is considered to be an essential one among well-known citrus oils utilized in aromatherapy because it is a refreshing and tangy scent which can be very positive.

Essential oils of grapefruit are extremely healthy and beneficial for health due to the following characteristics:

Disinfectant.

Aperitif.

Antiseptic.

Diuretic.

Stimulant.

Antidepressant.

Lemon essential oil

Lemons are among the most well-known citrus fruits, and they are popular because they're an excellent source of vitamins and can help with digestion. The best thing about the essential oil of lemon is that it is nutritious, tasty and affordable. It is usually employed to ease stress due to its capacity to reenergize the mind. It also can be very relaxing. In terms of weight loss , it is a great choice because it reduces potential to reduce the effects of eating too much. It's rich in vitamin content and improves the immune system of the body. Essential oil of lemon is believed to possess the following qualities:

Anti-fungal.

Antioxidant.

Antidepressant.

Refreshing.

Antiseptic.

Antiviral.

Invigorating.

Tonic.

Bergamot essential oil

Bergamot essential oil produced by hand or cold pressing the skin of the ripe fruit of the Bergamot tree. The bergamot tree is made by crossing the lemon with that of the orange trees. The essential oil of bergamot contains flavoinoids that make it vital as a relaxing agent. They also play a significant role in relieving nerve tension as well as reducing tension in the nervous system and and stress control. It aids digestion because it stimulates the release of enzymes, digestive acids, and the bile. The entire concept behind being able to assist in overcoming anxiety and depression by reducing stress comes from its fresh and refreshing citrus scent. Bergamot essential oil is known to have the following qualities:

Antibiotic.

Antiseptic.

Antispasmodic.

Antidepressant.

Sedative.

Disinfectant.

Vulnerary.

Lavender essential oil

Essential oils of lavender have been since the beginning of time to aid in healing and religious purposes. It is extracted by steam distillation using flowers from the plant. Lavender essential oil can have an euphoric and relaxing affect on the body. this helps heal emotionally and physically. It is highly efficient and is an essential oil that aids in getting better sleep as well as healing burns and injuries and anxiety, as well as reducing anxiety and depression. Essential oil of lavender is believed to have following properties:

Antimicrobial.

Antidepressant.

Anti-fungal.

Antibacterial.

Analgesic.

Sedative.

Detoxifying.

Peppermint essential oil

The essential oils of peppermint are a cross species that combines spearmint and watermint . It is also extracted by steam distillation. It is among the oldest essential oils that provides a cooling sensation and has a relaxing and soothing effects on the body. It assists in improving concentration as well as easing stomachaches. improves energy levels, reduces headaches, relaxes muscles, reduces stress, and decreases cravings for food. The essential oil peppermint is believed to have following properties:

Antibacterial.

Antiseptic.

Analgesic.

Antiviral.

Anti-inflammatory.

Invigorating.

Cypress essential oil

Cypress essential oil is generally made by steam distillation process of young twigs needles, and stems. Recently, cypress oil is widely used in both medicinal and industrial usage. It is applied by massage and inhalation. The benefits of cypress essential oil is it eases discomfort, relaxes the nerve system, and strengthens and tightens the tissues and reduces blood vessel constrictions. It is completely safe for use and is non-toxic. However, it is advised to conduct a skin patch test prior to applying it on the skin. It's also believed to be a good blend with other oils that are woody e.g. pine oil and cedarwood oil. The aroma of the oil can help people who are weak and emotionally unstable. The essential oil of Cypress is believed to possess the following qualities:

Diuretic.

Antiseptic.

Sedative.

Astringent.

Tonic for the respiratory tract.

Antispasmodic.

Deodorant.

Basil essential oil

The oil of basil is rich food source for vitamin A, potassium magnesium, iron and calcium. It is often employed in cooking since it tastes delicious and increases the flavor and aroma in your meal. Inhaling basil oil helps to refresh the mind and sharpens your concentration. The traditional use of basil oil was to help support the respiratory system, and digestion through inhaling the powdered leaves. Since it is an energizing and energizing oil, it' most effective in the morning and during the daytime. Basil essential oil has been believed to possess the following properties

Antibacterial.

Antispasmodic.

Uplifting.

Diuretic.

Antioxidant.

Disinfectant.

Stimulant.

Cinnamon essential oil

It is used extensively to flavor food and for medicinal use. It is also believed for causing allergic reactions and irritations However, it does have numerous health advantages. It helps in boosting brain activity, blood purification, pain relief, ingestion etc. its properties aid in boosting immunity since it promotes an active and healthy cardiovascular system. While the powder of cinnamon is safe to consume, cinnamon leaf oil shouldn't be used internally without medical supervision. It is recommended to use it in moderation, and only after appropriate dilution since high doses may cause convulsions for some individuals. Essential oil of cinnamon is believed to possess the following properties:

Antibacterial.

Anti-fungal.

Antiseptic.

Antimicrobial.

Antidepressant.

Antioxidant.

Antispasmodic.

Purifier.

Anti-inflammatory.

Oregano essential oil

The essential oil is made from fresh oregano leaves by steam distillation. It is a potent source of health benefits, however it is mostly linked to respiratory health and your immune system. It is therefore helpful in the treatment of infections of the respiratory tract, urinary tract yeast infections as well as parasitic infections. As long as you dilute it with water or in carrier oil, oregano oil is safe for use. However, you must still conduct an exam on your skin to confirm that you're not in any way allergic. It is possible to take fresh or dried oregano, but the oil is more efficient and beneficial. Oregano essential oil has been believed to possess the following qualities:

Antibacterial.

Anti-fungal.

Digestive.

Antiviral.

Antioxidant.

Anti-inflammatory.

Anti-parasitic.

Rosemary essential oil

The essential oil of rosemary is extracted from the rosemary plant mostly by removing the leaf of Rosmarinus Officianalis. It is utilized to treat ailments at home and for medicinal use. It has a sweet scent that has the ability to alter the mood of a person, causing them to become more aware and alert. In addition to being used in hair and skin care products, rosemary essential oil can have health benefits such as improving memory, relieving pain, eases anxiousness and nerves, and increases blood circulation. When the rosemary oil massaged on the back of an individual, it could aid in strengthening and protecting the nerves. The essential oil of rosemary is believed to possess the following properties:

Antibacterial.

Anti-fungal.

Antioxidant.

Anticancer.

Anti-inflammatory.

Anti-infections.

Chapter 6: Mistakes To Avoid

There are many mistakes you could make, particularly in the beginning stages of beginning to explore your options using essential oils. This chapter will provide you with some basics to look out for when making use of essential oils. If you adhere to these guidelines the experience you have with essential oils can be more relaxing.

Be sure to follow all Safety Recommendations

Even though essential oils are organic doesn't mean they are 100% safe. There are guidelines for their use you must follow for example:

Keep oil away from children.

Do not get the oils or other products made from oils to your eyes.

Test a patch on a small portion of your face to make sure you're not allergic to the oil or any product that you create.

Make sure you take extra precautions if are nursing, pregnant or using the oils on your children. Review the oil's instructions to use them in these scenarios.

Speak with a professional prior to you are using oils internally, such as an experienced physician or aromatherapist.

Certain essential oils can trigger your skin's ability to turn phototoxic. Avoid exposure to sunlight when applying the oils applied topically.

Check to see if oils can work against one or create unwanted negative side effects when used combination.

Decreased Sensitization to Oils

If you apply the identical essential oils for a long time it will eventually reduce their effectiveness. It is because you become numb to their effects. This is the reason it's recommended to keep some essential oils are used for various purposes. For instance, there are several oils mentioned in this guide that assist in suppressing appetite. If one of them fails to work for you, then try another. This will allow you to get the long-term results you're looking for.

Mix Oils into the Bath

When essential oils are added into the tub they will be placed on high-end of the tub. If you're sensitized to essential oils or are using them for children make sure to mix the essential oil and an oil carrier to avoid sensitization from bathing.

Don't Buy Cheap

A lot of people are looking to reduce expenses This is normal. But anything you put on your body or put in it must be of top quality. It is therefore essential to buy the finest oils you can get. Be sure they've been tested and confirmed as to be pure. If you plan to take the oils internally, that you are getting foods grade oils only. Be sure that the other oils you buy are therapeutic quality. Purchase your oils in a pure form and create the rubs, salts and other products. If you purchase oil that is mixed then you do not really know what the oils are made of and it might not be beneficial to you.

Ask Questions

It is essential to have any questions you may have about essential oils. The book offers a basic overview, but it might not provide all the information you're seeking to learn about. Making contact with a qualified aromatherapist could be among the most beneficial things is possible to do. Additionally, you can ask the suppliers of the products you purchase any questions you might have about the products you're purchasing. This can help you save more money if avoid buying items that aren't needed.

When purchasing essential oils, there are certain questions you need to inquire about, for instance:

Are your oils certified organic? (Only make use of organic oils to treat.)

Are these oils safe to consume?

Have your oils been examined to ensure they're potent and contain no added ingredients?

Are your oils being tested by a third-party to ensure that they're doing the job you've promised them to do?

Are you able to visit the farms where plants are grown to produce the oils you use? Are you confident about their sustainability and the quality of their oil?

Learn as much as you Are Able To

This book is a fantastic starting point to use essential oils to shed pounds, but you might want to think about adding more essential oils to your routine. Learn a class, buy additional books, and speak to those who have been who are trained to use essential oils. It's a complex subject that has many avenues to learn. This book will teach you the basic information you need to begin however there's many more details available. Do not be afraid to look into the subject.

Be sure to handle your Oils in a safe manner

Many people who aren't familiar with essential oils don't treat oils with the care they require. In the previous section, we covered how to store and handle your oils. If you don't follow these guidelines the oils won't keep their beneficial effects. Many individuals choose to purchase the oils they need in smaller quantities to ensure they don't lose their effectiveness. Be sure to follow the storage tips within the FAQ section to ensure the most effective outcome when the storage of oils.

Do Not Apply Oils All Over Your Body on Your Body

If oils can be applied to the body, it is usually specifically outlined as to the best place to apply it and the frequency of use. Oils shouldn't be spread all on your body. Also, you should be aware whether the oils can increase your vulnerability to sunburn.

It is possible to overdose on Essential Oils

Always follow the instructions for using the oils. A prolonged usage of an oil could result in an overdose. Keep in mind that all natural products come with specific instructions for their use. The guidelines in this publication for particular oils that are used to reduce weight, as well as the information contained on the bottles you purchase must be followed. In the absence of following these guidelines, you can lead to a variety of problems.

Don't Quit!

If an essential oil doesn't suit your needs, consider a different one. Similar to medication, not all essential oils will perform exactly in the same way for all individuals. The concept of bio-individuality present, meaning that what is effective for someone else could not work for you. As we've said previously, there are a variety of different oils that can produce the same results and it's worthwhile to experiment and find out which one works best for you.

Chapter 7: Combining Essential Oils

There are two reasons essential oils are paired in order to gain greater benefits as well as to produce an aroma that is more pleasing.

To receive additional benefits

It's sometimes easier to mix several essential oils that are utilized for different reasons to eliminate the need to apply various products separately. For instance, if someone is looking to get rid of dark spots on the skin for a more uniform skin tone and also to boost blood flow to keep youthful appearance you can apply rose essential oil that can be used for both. But, if the person is not a fan of the smell of roses, she could make use of a blend of lavender and lemon. Instead of using the two essential oils in isolation it's more practical to combine them in equal quantities and keep the solution in an additional container.

To give a enjoyable smell

It's possible that you get bored of using one essential oil with its distinctive scent. Hence it's a great idea to make a new scent.

Mixing essential oils to create an aroma that is different is not straightforward. Professional perfumers have to learn for a while before they are able to get their recipe correct, but novices can experiment with these easy scent combinations:

1:1 lemon and lavender

1:1 rose + sandalwood

2:2:1 roses, sandalwood and vanilla

1:1 vanilla, jasmine and vanilla

2:2:1 rosemary, peppermint , and grapefruit

Note, however it is important to note that when using essential oils to treat aromatherapy, i.e. getting all the advantages of oils by inhaling their scents, the combined essential oils will offer a multitude of advantages. Vanilla for example is relaxing, while jasmine boosts concentration. This could be a great mix for people who have been anxious and struggle to focus, but it's not a great combination for those suffering from insomnia as jasmine could make them sleepy.

Additional details about essential oil recipes for fragrance can be found in websites and books about fragrances.

While discussing Aromatherapy, we noted at the beginning of chapter one that premium synthetic fragrance oils may be substituted for essential oils. They are cheaper than real essential oils and smell exactly like real oils however, discerning noses and those familiar with the smell of genuine essential oils could be able detect an underlying difference.

In no way should inexpensive artificial fragrance oils be employed. They are readily available at a bargain and may cost less than $1 per bottle, and are found in the home décor section of a lot of discount shops. These scents tend to trigger headaches than to provide any benefits.

Chapter 8: Essential Oils for Personal Care Recipes

Alongside weight loss and mood-lifting blends, blends of essential oils may be made for cosmetic reasons. They can be utilized as anti-aging treatments, and to improve the appearance of your hair, and skin.

If the carrier oil you're using is, such as jojoba or olive oil It is recommended to mix the carrier oil with the other essential ingredients at least a few days prior to before you use the oils. So the ingredients get an opportunity to settle and blend thoroughly prior to using. Here are some ideas you can try right now to improve your appearance and overall well-being.

Aromatic Blend for general skin care:

To get glowing young skin, mix one quarter cup of olive or almond oil along with 10 drops of lavender and the rosewood oil 10 drops along with 10 drops of oil from sandalwood.

Combine the ingredients and apply it to the skin areas you want to improve. This can be done every all day or every once in time.

Essential Oil Mixture to Get Free of Corns:

To soothe your feet and enhance their appearance Mix two ounces almond or olive oil with six drops myrrh essential oil as well as the essential oils of 12 lavender drops.

Mix the oils in a bottle, then apply it to the areas you need. Make use of this mixture daily until the corns go away off your feet.

A Blend to Soften Calluses

Two tablespoons of almond oil or olive oil to make the base. Then add 20 drops of lavender oil. Add 5 drops of the carrot seeds and 10 drops of the chamomile oil.

Mix them in a bottle before applying on the calluses at least twice per daily. To make it more effective soak the areas of calluses and then rub them to aid in the removal of hardened skin. Pumice stones can help to make this more effective. After getting rid of your calluses, continue making this mixture often to prevent them from coming back.

An Skin Toning Mixture

To make this recipe, make use of eight ounces of distillated water for the base, and then you will add 1 drop of each palmarosa and rosewood oils and 2 drops lavender oils.

Mix it all up in a glass bottle , and shake vigorously to mix. Apply the mixture to the desired areas with the help of a cotton ball. Each time you decide to apply this mix shake it up again. It is possible to use it at least once per day depending on the need.

A Rejuvenating Blend for face care:

Make use of 1 tablespoon olive oil to make the base of this mix. Add 2 drops of lavender, and one drop of Geranium.

Combine the ingredients and apply the mixture to the face following washing. The mixture can be applied at least once per day.

Blend of Facial Oil to eliminate skin Dryness:

Make use of oil like olive, jojoba, or almond oil for the base. Mix 1 tablespoon of your preferred carrier oils with an ounce of chamomile oil and two drops of neroli oil.

Mix them together and apply it to your skin after you've washed. It can be applied whenever you need to and 2 times per every day is recommended. It's an ideal idea to mix essential oils and carrier oil two days in advance so that the oils can get a solid foundation.

A Young Serum for aging skin:

Almond oil is suggested to be the primary carrier oil in this recipe. Mix one tablespoon of almond oil with two drops of Frankincense Oil, and 1 drop rose oil.

Mix them in a glass container and apply it to your face to rehydrate and revive tired skin. It is also possible to apply moisturizing creams for face avocado oil, avocado oil, or olive oil in place in place of almond oil.

Formula for Healthy Lungs:

To make this mix, boil two cups of pure water. In another container, mix six drops of the oils of cedarwood and peppermint 3 drops of rosemary along with 12 drops Eucalyptus oil.

Mix the oils inside a bottle of glass, then shake the bottle to mix. Pour your boiling water into the stainless-steel bowl. Then, add around 5 drops oil to 2 cups water. Place your head on the bowl, and then place the help of a towel to inhale the steam through the mixture.

Homemade Body Powder for the Body:

Make use of two tablespoons of corn starch to form the base of this mix and mix it in with five drops of clove oil and spearmint and 10 drops of each of peppermint and spruce oil.

This mixture is able to be applied on your skin at any time you require to refresh yourself. Apply it to your body after bathing to keep you feeling healthy throughout the day.

A Skin Care Blend:

Take a quarter cup avocado, jojoba or almond oil for the carrier oil. After that, include 10 drops sandalwood, lavender and rosewood oils.

Mix these ingredients in a glass bottle , and use every day for facial maintenance.

Helps to fight oily hair:

The grapeseed oil makes the most suitable carrier oil to make this mix. Mix two tablespoons in nine drops of lime oil , and oil. Add 8 drops rosemary.

Mix the oils together and apply a tablespoon of the mixture to your hair one at a time. Massage the oil into your scalp and allow it to sit for a couple of hours. You can do this several times per week however, be certain that you wash hair afterward with a non-scented, chemical-free shampoo at least at least twice.

Detangling Spray-on Hair Conditioner

Make use of distilled water as the basis for this recipe. Mix 150mls of it with 5ml of an oil emulsifier, 20 drops oil of rosemary, 20 drops carrotseed oil as well as twenty drops lavender.

Mix the components in spray bottles, and shake vigorously to mix the ingredients. This is a great option for either dry or hair that is wet after showering. If you are using dry hair, spray it with enough to leave your hair slightly damp and then gently comb it. This will help to condition your hair and rid it of knots, leaving no unpleasant leftovers. If you have trouble in battling frizz then this product will aid with it too. It's soft enough to use each time you wash your hair. It can also be used prior to or after washing.

Relief for the Athletes Foot or Odor of the Foot Odor:

Make use of two ounces olive, jojoba or avocado oil for an oil base. Add six drops of each of myrrh and thyme oils along with the addition of eight drops of eucalyptus oil and the tea tree oils of 10 drops.

Mix all the ingredients together in a jar or bottle and shake it to mix. This mix may be applied on your feet as often as twice every day, as required. While the results will not be immediate but they should be visible in a matter of days. The more consistent you are in taking it, the more it'll be. Although relief from symptoms may be quick but it is highly recommended to use this product for a couple of weeks to eliminate all trace of infection and stop it from returning.

The formula for healing dry skin:

Mix 1 teaspoon of camellia oils, one teaspoon of olive oil or Jojoba oil, 1 teaspoon sesame oils two drops of Geranium, four drops neroli, six drops sandalwood and 25 drops carrotseed oil.

Combine all the ingredients above into the glass bottle and shake. You can use up to 6 drops of the blend to the desired areas of your skin up couple of times a every day. You will start noticing a difference quite quickly.

How to Stop Hair Loss:

For this recipe , you will require one tablespoon of jojoba oil 1 tablespoon of olive or almond oil 40 drops carrotseed oil, 10 , drops lavender four drops each of lavender and rosemary, as well as six drops of clary-sage.

Mix the above ingredients in a jar or bottle with a lid, and shake to mix. Then, head the ingredients prior to applying the mix to your head. take a couple of drops at each time. The solution can be left for a few hours , or for a night time period using the use of a shower cap. It can be used at least once a week, or whenever necessary.

A Blend to Help Relieve sunburned skin:

For this blend , you'll require two ounces of jojoba oil and distilled water. Include sixty drops of lavender oil, and 25 drops of Helichrysum.

Combine all the ingredients above in a spray bottle made of plastic and apply it to the irritated, sunburned skin as frequently as is necessary. To store, keep it out from the sun in a cool location.

Mix for perfume:

This recipe will require 1 ounce of Jojoba Oil and 25 drops vanilla oil 5 drops of each clove and rose oils 10 drops of each of

Clary safe, bergamot and lavender, as well as 20 drogs of Helichrysum.

Mix all of the ingredients in the container of your choice and allow the mix to blend for 7 days. It may be used in very small doses to hair or the skin to create a pleasant smell.

An Acne and oily Skin Cure:

There are the following ingredients: four cups boiling water four drops of oil from cypress, the oil of a lemon, four drops along with six drops of Juniper to prepare this recipe.

Combine all the oils mentioned above in one cup, and mix them together. Take the freshly heated water and put it in the bowl. Incorporate the oils into the bowl, and then place an over-the-head towel. Lean over the bowl and let the steam be absorbed by your face. Give it five minutes before washing it off with cool water. Dry by gently rubbing it using the towel. This will help to treat your skin issues. It can be done every week or once depending on the need.

Foot Deodorizing Powder:

One tablespoon baking soda will be the basis, together with two ounces Talc powder. Then you can add two drops of spearmint, sage and coriander.

Take the lid off of the container of talc powder, and add the teaspoon of baking soda. Mix thoroughly by shaking the contents. To make use of the oils that come with this powder, simply add drops onto a cotton ball. put the cotton ball into the powder bottle. Allow to mix for two days prior to using. It is possible to apply it directly on your feet or apply it to on the soles of shoes.

Oil for Beating Wrinkles:

To make this blend, you'll require 10 drops of primrose, carrotseed, lemon, fennel lavender, neroli and oil, as well as 3 drops rosemary as well as two teaspoons hazelnut or almond oil.

Mix all the ingredients in a glass bottle , then shake it to mix the ingredients. It can be applied to your face and neck each night when you wash your face. For primrose oil to be used to use, you'll have to buy gel capsules , then cut them open in order to get the oil. The reason for this is that you require a tiny amount.

Chapter 9: Why Do Essential Oils Some of the Most Important?

More Effective than Other?

Much of it is related to the manufacturing process, but some of it is related to environmental.

On the other hand, environmental factors it is possible for almost anything to affect the therapeutic potential of essential oils. Factors like geography, climate soil conditions and the altitude at which the initial plant was harvested may alter how much oil it creates.

This is due to the fact that chemical components change in response to changing conditions.

Essential oil producers influence the therapeutic benefits of their oil. The characteristics of the plant vary based on the season of harvest as well as whether or the fertilizer used to cultivate the plant was organic and even the process of distillation (which involves choosing the part of the plant to which oil to extract)

Thyme is a plant that produces a variety of chemical compounds (biochemical particulars) dependent on the conditions under which it grows. If it is distilled during the fall or mid-summer the plant will produce more carvacrol, which can cause irritation to your skin.

How to Mix

Essential Oils

Since essential oils are concentrated, they could be dangerous when consumed by themselves.

A few essential oils can be used undiluted and, even then it is recommended to use them in small amounts. They include Lavender, German Chamomile, Tea Tree, Sandalwood, and Rose Geranium.

Pure essential oils must be mixed in conjunction with carriers oils (like alcohols, waxes or any other diluting substances) prior to using them.

This is actually a good thing because, even though pure essential oils can be expensive however, only a small amount of them actually need to be utilized to achieve the desired result.

When choosing the right carrier oil is important to be aware about the fats contained in this substance. While they're generally good for the body, they might not be ideal for essential oils and could cause faster rancidity (which is actually the fancy term for decay).

The most common rule of thumb in the case of mixing essential oils and a carrier oil goes as follows:

The Measurements/Conversions by Volume, as it pertains to essential oil dilution with carrier oils:

30 ml = 1 fl oz = 600 drops = 2 tablespoons

15 ml = 1/2 fl oz = 300 drops = 1 tablespoon

5 milliliters = 1/6 fl. 1 oz = 100 drops equals 1 teaspoon

1 milliliter = 1/30 fl. oz = 20 drops equals 1/5 teaspoon

To get a certain dilution, here's an equation that will make it easy to determine the amount of drops you should use per fluid ounce

To get one fluid (1 1 oz) one ounce of Carrier Oil:

1percent of 600 drops (1 1 fl 1 oz) equals 6 drops

2.2 percent from 600 drops (1 1 fl 1 oz) equals 12 drops

2.5 percent out of the 600 drops (1 1 fl. 1 oz) equals 15 drops

5percent of 600 drops (1 1 fl 1 oz) equals 30 drops

10 percent out of the 600 drops (1 1 fl 1 oz) equals 60 drops

It is crucial to follow the instructions to any recipe once you begin mixing essential oils and carrier oils. Also in the event that the recipe is intended to be administered to children, reduce the quantity of essential oils included in the recipe by half. Children have thinner, less delicate skin than adults and the traditional recipes could be too strong for them.

Never use essential oil that has not been diluted for children or babies.

Pure essential oils can be around 70x more powerful than total plant. The typical dilution is between 2% and 10 percent. For adults the recommended dosage is 2.5 percent dilution is suggested for the majority of uses. For children who are less than 12 years old, 1percent is considered to be safe. A 2.5 percentage blend for a one-ounce bottle contains fifteen drops essential oils.

Blend of 1% equals 6 drops per one ounce

A 2% blend equals 12 drops per one ounce

Blend of 3% equals 18 drops for each 1 oz

Blend of 5% = 30 drops per one oz

10 percent blend equals 60 drops per 1 oz

Keeping & Storing

Essential Oils

Another thing that could help lower the price of premium essential oils that are pure and of the highest quality is the longevity.

If properly maintained and properly maintained, essential oils are likely to last between 5 to 10 years. (The only exception to this is the citrus essential oils which lose their effectiveness after one year or as).

To make sure that your essential oils get the best chance to last for a long time, and keeping their potency, you need ensure that they are stored properly.

One reason is that sunlight can seriously damage essential oils over the course of time. Therefore, it is essential to keep them away from direct sunlight, preferably in an dark cabinet. It is also recommended to keep them in dark glass bottles (usually that they come packaged in appropriate bottles).

It also assists in keeping the oils in a cool zone. Low temperatures and low pressure aid in maintaining the purity, aroma and the therapeutic value of your essential oils.

Three exceptions exist to the principle, also: Sandalwood, Vetiver and Patchouli essential oils actually become better with time, much as the best wines.

For the carrier oils you use It is essential to store them refrigerated in airtight containers. This can help to avoid rancidity.

How to safely absorb

Essential Oils

Now that you have an a basic understanding of the essence of what Essential Oils are and how they're pure and how they can be stored and some guidelines on how they can be incorporated into carrier oils, it is time to look at the different methods to take them in.

There are many methods to accomplish this, and selecting the most appropriate method will depend on the benefits you're seeking.

It's not advisable even if you massage essential oils on your skin, if it is, for instance, the therapeutic benefits you're looking for is to treat respiratory issues.

Different methods work best for various oils, too. Certain oils can be taken in through the skin, while others must be consumed in order to benefit from their properties.

Dosages may also differ based on the method of absorption employed.

Below is an overview of the different ways to use essential oils. Be sure to research more about the particular oil you're using, and speak with a doctor for any health concerns before diving into any holistic cure.

Also, remember that it is inappropriate for women who are pregnant to apply essential oils without talking to their doctor first.

Inhalation

If you're seeking relief of headaches, or sinus issues The method is extremely beneficial. Inhaling essential oils through diffusers, in hot water (by breathing in steam) and also through hot compresses that are placed near your sinus region.

The most common dosage for this kind for absorption can be 10 drops. It is diluted by the boiling water and diffusion.

One aspect that must be considered, however it is only a temporary issue. The prolonged inhalation of essential oils can trigger nausea, headaches, vertigo and dizziness. Make sure you get away from the area and inhale fresh air whenever you notice some of these symptoms coming on.

It is also far not a cure for respiratory ailments that are chronic. It's for preventative treatment and temporary relief. If you suffer from asthma, do not use it as an all-time replacement for your inhaler that you can use as a rescue.

Baths

This particular method is an alternative approach to two of the techniques listed (direct-skin-contact as well as inhalation).

In order to disperse your oils in a safe manner in the water Mix your important oils in bathtub salts (pure Epsom salt works the best). Also, you can employ as an emulsifier (like milk or sesame oil as well as coconut oil).

If you do not mix the essential oils with the items that are listed, they'll appear in the form of tiny dots. They will not be diluted properly since essential oils aren't able to mix perfectly with water. This can lead to unsafe direct skin-to-skin contact.

This is a bigger problem if the oils are of a hot nature, such as Cinnamon Oil, Oregano Oil, Thyme Oil, or Tulsi Oil. Because, when they are combined with the warmth of your bathing water, they could be considered to be the skin's epitomizer (toxic on the health of your skin). This is also the case with citrus oils such as Bergamot Oil or Lemongrass Oil. In reality with the specific oils, it's better to utilize them in a different method (like treatments or other glandular techniques).

In order to avoid serious skin irritation, take our suggestions and mix the salts mentioned above with as well as carrier oils and milk.

There are numerous essential oils recommended to bathe with. They are Lavender Oil, Clary Sage Oil, Rose Oil, Geranium Oil, Frankincense Oil, Sandalwood Oil, and Eucalyptus Oil.

There are also Conifers (which are plants that contain seeds from a cone with a woody bracted) including Cedar Oil, Fir Oil, Pine Oil, Pinon Pine Oil, Spruce Oil as well as Juniper Oil.

Dosages for baths differ little however, it's generally recommended to use between 5 and 10 drops of essential oils for every 1/2-to-1 cup of salt or an emulsifier.

Essential oil massages are an excellent option to treat respiratory and circulatory problems as well as insomnia, muscular and menstrual cramps, as well as skin problems (like dry or acne-prone skin) as well as to relieve anxiety, stress, and tension.

It is crucial not to use too much essential oils baths. Typically, 1 to 2 essential oil baths each week is sufficient to reap the therapeutic benefits, without causing discomfort to the skin or vomiting.

Compresses

Essential oils are beneficial in the healing of minor wounds, bruises, dysmenorrhea, muscle pain and skin issues when they are applied in homemade compresses.

If you are suffering from bruises, you can add fresh sage and 10 drops lavender oil, and then 4 ounces hot water.

For all types of compresses, let the mixture get hot (don't make it boil, however) and then soak an unclean cloth in it for a couple of minutes. Then, take the cloth out of the mix and place it on the part you would like to heal.

The rest of the mix in an airtight container to ensure security and then place the container in the fridge for at least a day or two. It should be possible reuse it at least more times prior to throwing it away.

Facial Steams

One way to absorb essential oils is to make the use of a homemade facial steam. This is like the method of inhalation however it offers a greater direct contact with the vapors.

This is why it's recommended to reduce the dose to around half the amount you'd need to inhale normally (1-5 drops is sufficient).

Set a pot of boiling liquid on your stove to and heat it up (but don't let it boil) and add drops. Cover your head with an untidy towel (try to use a towel that has been washed using a detergent that isn't scented and/or non-scented softeners). Relax your body toward the pot, then let it rise and then hit your face.

This will open your sinuses, which can ease migraines and headaches. It's also a great method to unblock your pores , which will help nourish and cleanse your skin.

As with all inhalations make sure to take in fresh air when you begin feeling dizzy or nauseated. It's only necessary to perform this for up to one minute to get the desired results. Generally it's not even all that long.

Massages

The method of massage is fairly easy to explain. It's used to ease tension headaches, muscle pains and nervous tension. It's also good to improve skin tone and circulation in problematic areas when you are using essential oils that enhance cellular regeneration.

You can accomplish this with ease since essential oils are liptropic (which is to say they're fat-soluble) therefore they'll be absorbed by your skin in a matter of minutes.

Make sure to dilute essential oils correctly before letting them touch your skin. Carrier oils such as sweet grapeseed oil and almond oil are suggested since they're less viscous than oil that is thicker (like coconut oil or sesame oil) and are absorbed by the skin quicker.

Jasmine Oil, Neroli Oil, Rose Oil, Vanilla Oil and Marula Oil are great for massage oils.

It is also possible to use Citrus Oils at smaller amounts (1-3 drops for each ounce carrier oil) in order to revive your skin.

Direct Palm Inhalations

This is a form of deep inhalation that can only be used with very specific oils (the milder ones that are safe for direct-skin-contact.)

It's a quick-acting method to absorb the antimicrobial and therapeutic properties of essential oils. It's also great for treating migraines.

Because the oils won't be dilute, you will only require 1 or 2 drops to use this method.

Certain oils that are safe to use for the direct inhalation method include Lavender Oil, Clary Sage Oil, Rose Oil, Geranium Oil, Frankincense Oil, Sandalwood Oil as well as Eucalyptus Oil.

Diffusers

Diffusers are fantastic as they emit the advantages of essential oils while creating a wonderful scent for your home.

There are many ways to diffuse essential oils.

The Electric Heat Diffusers* are tiny absorbent pads placed in an air-conditioned heating chamber that allow the oil to evaporate to the air. They are simple to operate, need only minimal maintenance and are able of diffusing heavier oils. Be cautious when using these as some essential oils contain chemical compounds which change when they're heated. Avoid citrus oils such as Bergamot Oil as well as Lemongrass Oil when using this method.

Candle Diffusers comprise small, usually portable, heat-resistant container to store essential oils and water together with a durable heat-resistant platform that is used to support the vessel on top of a tiny candle. They're very simple to use and offer illumination as well as a pleasant scent, however they do not provide a high concentration of essential oils that you're seeking for benefits that are therapeutic.

Cool-Air Nebulizing Diffusers* make use of air pressure created by a compressor unit. This pressure in the air evaporates the essential oil, while the glass nebulizing lamp compresses the oils, which allows only the most effective particles of the essential oil to escape in the open air.

They're a good alternative to heat-operated diffusers when you're trying to make use of oils that are not compatible when heated up to high temperatures. They supply a large amount of essential oils, and, as a consequence they can be extremely beneficial (especially in respiratory issues such as asthma, bronchitis or sinus infections.)

The only thing to remember is that they must be regularly cleaned and can't disperse oils that are thicker like Sandalwood.

Cool air nebulizing diffusers

A device that utilizes the force of air created by a compressor unit to evaporate essential oils. Nebulizing bulbs made of glass serve as a condenser and allows only the most pure parts of the essence oil escape to the air.

It is essential to use an electronic timer and cool air Nebulizers. These products produce a greater concentration of essential oils. A timer can help you keep yourself from over-saturating.

Glandular

To get the most potent medicinal effects of essential oils it is possible to absorb them via blood circulation. If absorbed in this manner essential oils can also affect the olfactory pathways that connect your brain.

It is the most efficient method to treat sinus issues and neurological issues, migraines, emotional imbalances and immune-related issues since it affects the blood supply directly.

Patchouli oil is a great choice to take this kind of absorption since it stimulates your pituitary gland. It creates endorphins in a natural way that induce positive feelings and is an holistic painkiller.

The absorption of glandular oils can be accomplished via massage or by inhalation when you're in a room that is warm. The essential oils travel through sweat glands and hair follicles when you use the massage technique as well as through your airways and olfactory system through an inhalation technique.

When you're applying the method of massage you should put a little the mixture on areas where your skin is thin (like wrists, your temples and armpits, behind your ears or on your feet and palms) because it's more permeable and can soak up the essential oil faster.

The essential oil mix will be absorbed into the skin, then enter your capillaries, and eventually float across your bloodstream.

Consider it as a form of mainlining therapy that involves gentle massage.

Chapter 10: Uses And Benefits Of Essential Oils

The essential oils are utilized throughout history to promote physical, mental, and therapeutic well-being. Essential oils are used to treat aromatherapy, in cooking, to help reduce anxiety, stress, depression, as mood boosters and enhancing the function of the brain, boosting levels of energy, and as perfumes. Essential oils are a wealth of anti-bacterial, antiseptic, analgesic antioxidant, anti-inflammatory, and anti-oxidant properties. They can help digestion, to keep you healthy, offer relief from pain and also reduce swelling and itching from bites from insects. If you're suffering from cold or flu essential oils can help in the decongestion process and also aid in the ear infection. It is no secret that sleep is essential; various essential oils are known to can help you relax and sleep and help you sleep deeply so that you can wake up feeling rejuvenated and revived. The addition of flavorings to food can be a great method to utilize essential oils in addition to soothing irritation of the skin, a great supplement to shampoo and a room freshener. There's no end to the advantages!

The following list of suggestions outlines the beneficial ways you can make use of essential oils, with all their uses to improve physical and mental health, and to treat various illnesses.

All-purpose cleaner: Add 2 drops of tea tree and lemon oil to water and vinegar and use it for multi-purpose cleaning

Mosquito Repellant: Add 3 drops of citronella, lemon grass and eucalyptus, as well as 1 drop and 1 teaspoon of coconut oil

Cleaning Gym Clothes 2 drops of tea tree oil in large bowls of warm water. Then add 1/4 cup baking soda to mix. Allow to soak for 30 minutes.

Air Freshener 5 drops of rose oil and orange inside a spray bottle, or 10 drops in the diffuser

Cleansing clothes: Put 1 or 2 drops of your preferred essential oil to the washing machine to create a natural fragrance your clothes.

Sunscreen: mix equal parts of coconut oil, zinc oxide shea butter as well as 4 drops of lavender oil and helichrysum oil.

Kill Mold: To shower use Add 4 drops of tea tree oil. Spray down the shower. Alternatively, you can add 10 drops each in diffusers to remove the smell of mold.

Pan Scrubber: Add two drops of oil from a lemon to boiling water to get rid of stuck grease

Carpet Cleaner: Add four drops of tea oil from trees to Borax and mix it along with your carpet cleaner

Pest Control: Add 5 drops of clove and orange oil in a spray bottle that is equal parts alcohol (avoid the use of rubbing alcohol) and distillate water. Spray in areas where pests are or are living.

Wood or Fire Logs The best way to add some drops sandalwood, pine and cedar wood to your firewood or fire log for 30 minutes prior to burning

Reduce Stress and Anxiety: It is possible to use lavender with a spray bottle, or another recipe that is great for applying to the skin is to apply a few drops of lavender, chamomile and peppermint and unscented lotion applied to the your temples or on your hands

Increased Concentration Ten drops of Frankincense in the diffuser

Bath Cleaner: Mix 1/2 cup baking soda half cup of vinegar and 5 drops lime or bergamot oil

Trash can Use a cotton ball to soak in tea tree oil, and then place it in a trash container or in the back of a trash bin to help freshen the air.

Wash fruits and vegetables Mix 2 drops of oil from lemons into the large bowl of water, then wash your fruits and veggies in the bowl.

Bath Freshener: Dip the cotton ball in your preferred scent and put it behind the toilet to make an air freshener

Refrigerator Cleaner: add couple of drops of lime, grapefruit, and bergamot in warm water for cleaning.

Eliminate smoke Odors Incorporate 3 to 5 drops of rosemary, tea tree oil, and Eucalyptus oil to an aerosol bottle and spray the area where the odors originate.

Painting Mix 3 drops of peppermint as well as Eucalyptus to the paint containers to help reduce the odors

Freshening your shoe: To revive shoes , add 2 drops of tea tree oil per shoe. lemon and tea tree oil

Colic/Sleep Aid for Babies Apply 1 drop of lavender or the oil of chamomile to your hands, and allow your baby to breathe the oil between 12 and 18 inches from their face. It is also possible to add some drops of lavender and chamomile to baby's stuffed animals.

Dish Washer Use the oil of a lemon 2 drops in the dishwasher for clean as well as sparkling dishes!

Sleeping disorders You can sprinkle a few drops of lavender onto your pillow to ensure an enjoyable night's sleep and assist in staying asleep the entire night.

Body Lotion: Mix equal amounts of coconut oil, shea butter with the equivalent of 3 drops from your preferred oil

Natural Lip Gloss/Chapped Lips: Mix coconut oil and beeswax with some drops of lavender oil

Bath Make sure to add to your bath your essential oils of choice like such as lavender (promote relaxation) and Bergamot (reduce anxiety) cinnamon/clove (energy) and rose oils (depression) and Epsom salt, or sea salt

Aching Feet Get the juice of a lemon oil or eucalyptus oil into the bath for a relaxing soak to ease tired feet

Yoga/Pilates practice Mix 8-10 drops of lavender and sandalwood into diffusers to aid in centering you while practicing the yoga and Pilates practice. You can also cleanse your yoga mat with some drops of clove oil, citrus oil, along with warm water.

Cellulite Treatment: Add 5 drops grapefruit juice to two teaspoons coconut oil. Then rub it over the affected area.

Perfume: Apply 1 drop of jasmine oil or lavender oil, vanilla oil for ladies and clove and cypress oil for men onto the neck and wrists (test the area before applying on your skin or diluting it initially)

Acne Control Acne Control: Mix 3 drops tea tree oil with 1 teaspoon of honey. apply the mixture to face with circular movements of your hands and rinse off

A fresh breather: one drop peppermint oil on your tongue (not recommended if not tried it before talk to an aromatherapist)

Natural Shampoo: Mix 2-3 drops of rosemary and lavender oil with equal parts Aloe Vera and Coconut Milk and baking soda. This remedy will last between 2 to 4 weeks

Sugar/Salt Scrub: For use for body care, mix 2 drops almond oil and equal parts of rock salt, and Himalayan sugar

Toothpaste: Add small however equal amounts, of baking soda, sea salt coconut oil, xylitol (caution warning: toxic to dogs) as well as 1 drop peppermint oil (or orange oil for children!)

Body spray Use 5-10 drops of your preferred essential oil scent into the spray bottle and spray your body immediately after bath or shower.

Hair Thickener Make sure to add some drops of oil from rosemary in your shampoo

Dandruff Treatment: To reduce dandruff and smooth your scalp, apply the lavender oil and ceder wood oil and basil oil to three tablespoons coconut oil. allow to sit for 10 minutes

Strong Nails Strong Nails: Add the equivalent of 10 drops of cinnamon essential oil, myrrh oil, and lemon oil 2 tablespoons vitamin E. After that, apply the rub to cuticles

To lessen wrinkles, add three drops of sandalwood oils, geranium oils lavender oil and frankincense oil the unscented lotion for your face.

Whiten Teeth: Mix the juice of 1 lemon up to 1/2 teaspoon coconut oil, and 1 fresh strawberry. Then rub the mixture onto teeth using fingers. Rinse after two minutes.

Stretch Marks Make a mixture of five drops of Frankincense oil the grapefruit oil and myrrh and coconut oil, and apply it on the affected areas

Face Mask/Scrub: Mix 1/4 cup yogurt, 1 cup of cornmeal with five drops of patchouli oil as well as grapefruit oil and lavender oil. You can use this as a facial scrub or put it on your face for 5-10 minutes and use as a face mask.

Reduce dark spots on the face: Mix 3 drops of the frankincense essential oil, lemon oil, lavender oil, test a tiny spot on the skin prior application; the best results are achieved when applied directly to the skin. consult an aromatherapist

Hair Mask: Mix 15 drops rosewood oil, five drops of oil from sandalwood as well as 5 drops lavender oil. make the mixture hot by placing it in an plastic bag or glass jar , and then submerge it with hot water to ensure the oil is warm then massage it into your hair, and leave for 20 minutes. After that, wash hair

Hair with oily hair Apply 10 drops of ylang-ylang oil, lime oil as well as rosemary oil, to two ounces unscented oil. Apply it 3-4 times per week

Dry, flaky feet Apply 2 drops of lavender oil to 2 tablespoons of coconut oil, and apply it to the feet's bottom. apply the mixture prior to going to going to bed. After that, put socks on feet. Wake up to feet that are smooth and fresh!

Nausea/Vomiting Inhale some drops of essential oils of ginger, peppermint as well as lavender oil, to your hand towel and breathe in to help reduce nausea and vomiting.

Migraine: Mix two drops lavender oil with peppermint oil. Apply to the temples and/or the the neck's back.

Coughs and congestion A few drops of Eucalyptus oil in an oil diffuser or hot water and use the steam that rises to clear your sinuses and chest.

Burns To treat burns, add some drops of lavender oil in aloe vera , and apply it to burns

Bug bites Apply lavender oil on insect bites to lessen itching and encourage healing.

Healthy Digestion A couple of drops of peppermint oil, ginger oil and fennel oils to your favorite beverage or drink

Bronchitis or Asthma support Make five drops of Eucalyptus oil peppermint oil and coconut oil into diffusers, then place it near you and breathe deeply. Alternatively, you could also add them to a towel to breathe deeply into the towel.

Aid in reducing bruises Heal Apply five drops of lavender, frankincense and 5 drops in 4 ounces water and apply it to bruises

Enhance the function of your brain: apply the hand of a towel, or place in a diffuser, couple of drops of Bergamot oils, grapefruit oil or peppermint oil. Then inhale throughout the day.

Menstrual Cramps Mix some drops of basil oil, sage oil and rosemary oil with unscented oils and apply to an absorbent towel. Apply to the abdomen. Let it sit for 5 to 10 minutes.

Psoriasis and Eczema: Combine lavender oil with shea butter and apply it to the affected area.

Healthy Circulation Healthy Circulation: Add 10 drops of grapefruit oil in the bath and allow to soak for at minimum 20 minutes

Hangovers: Mix six drops each of the oils such as juniper berry oil grapefruit oil, cedarwood oil, lavender oil lemon oil, and rosemary oil in the bath

Balance Blood Sugar/Suppress Appetitive Take the drops of peppermint as well as cinnamon oil on your hands or a hand towel, and then inhale

Reduce the effects of fatigue by inhaling peppermint oil to get an instant boost

Ringworm: Add 3 drops tea tree oils with coconut oil and apply it twice each day.

Head Lice: Mix 3 drops of lavender oil, thyme oil and Eucalyptus to 1 cup of unscented oil. apply it to the scalp and leave for 30 mins.

Poison Oak/Ivy drops of peppermint in unscented oil, and apply it to the the affected area.

Morning Sickness: Add some drops of lemon, lemon and ginger on an old towel. Take many deep breaths until nausea is gone

Aches in the neck and back Mix the caypress oil, peppermint oil along with ginger oil and cayenne coconut oil and pepper. apply it to stiff and sore muscles.

The most commonly used essential oils

You can clearly see, there are numerous benefits to essential oils. There are many essential oils that are used in the various recipes mentioned previously. There are many essential oils that are utilized frequently in essential oil recipes as well as for a myriad of illnesses. The most well-known essential oils to use is Roman Chamomile because it offers many advantages, including relaxing muscles, reducing menstrual cramps and cramps, as well as sedative properties, reduces depression and anxiety, aids fight insomnia, is soothing for children and acts for anti-inflammatory properties. It's easy to see the reason this essential oil is extremely popular! Below is a list of the most well-known essential oils and their advantages.

Clary Sage: prevents/reduces muscle spasms and cramps in menstrual cycles. It also reduces menstru as well as aphrodisiac effects, and promotes peaceful emotions and reduces anxiety and can even aid in labor by decreasing the pain

Eucalyptus is a wonderful essential oil to boost the immune system and help in fighting common colds decongestant, antiviral, stimulating and decongestant

Frankincense: This essential oil can also help support the immune system and calms rough and irritated skin by encouraging cell regeneration and growth

Ginger is known to promote digestive health, reduces constipation and gas, helps reduce nausea , vomiting and constipation. It also improves metabolism, and has anti-inflammatory properties.

Lavender soothes and calms helps reduce anxiety, and promotes healing, soothes insect bites. It also aids in general skin care and aids in the process of cell regeneration.

Lemon: antibacterial, anti-viral bug repellant and antimicrobial and a great product for cleaning.

Peppermint reduces nausea, it is an analgesic (reduces the pain) for sore and stiff muscles, assists in headache reduction and it can be energizing (not advised for children less than three years of age)

Rose: stimulates cell renewal It soothes the emotions and encourages feelings of happiness and joy It reduces stress and anxiety It also helps reduce symptoms of PMS

Rosemary is great for sinusitis, nasal congestion, respiratory congestion Expectorant, energizing and stimulates circulation

Tea Tree is antibacterial, antimicrobial and antifungal properties. and boosts the immune system.

Ylang ylang reduces muscles spasms, relaxes and calms it, decreases depression and is an aphrodisiac.

Each essential oil can be used as a stand-alone or in the combination of many oils that treat or aid in specific ailments that are unique to the conditions you suffer from. Add drops of the oil into a bath, add them in a diffuser, put the oils in a foot soak then apply it to your the skin, or use them in your body creams and facial lotions. Each of essential oils can be used as a stand-alone and offer a variety of benefits. They are also wallet comfortable.

Chapter 11: Fantastic Or Hocus Pocus? What is the best way to use essential oils?

You know the essence oils however, what can you do with them? You can buy a bottle and drink the whole thing while watching the magical potion do its work. Of course not.

The most important thing to consider with the essential oil is its aromatherapy that uses natural oils and scents to ease aches and burns, aches and mental dissonance, stress and other symptoms of metal to assist in keeping your body to a more balanced and healthy state. In order to achieve this you must incorporate essential oils to your everyday routine and make use of them to the maximum extent possible.

There are three different ways the essential oils could be utilized and the choice is based on two aspects such as the cause and how the oil should be utilized. There are oils you shouldn't rub on your skin, however, they are safe to breathe. Other oils you'd like to swallow however, they are a bit unpleasant to smell. There isn't a single trick that solution to all problems here. It's a good combination that requires a thorough understanding of the best ways to utilize these techniques.

Luckily, many essential oils come with instructions on the bottle. You're probably buying the oils from someone else, and you can ask for assistance when you're unsure.

The most common method you could make use of essential oil is to inhale the oils. There are some selling essential oils have begun making small capsules that look like similar to the odd kind of fish eyes or mints. The capsules break down upon placing their contents on the tongue. The capsules are swallowed in order to ensure you get the oil right away to relieve discomfort in your stomach or pains within your throat. There are many oils that can aid you to fight off illnesses such as flu or colds.

Additionally, there are essential oils that come in droppers and are added to drinks like tea or coffee that you could drink to help get the oil in your body as quickly as possible.

Another method you could utilize essential oils in your present situation is to apply the oil as a lotion and apply it to the affected part. This is an excellent option to ease breathing and pains that you experience within your body.

Make sure you're using only oils that are guaranteed to be used for physical contact. It's important to be aware of the amount of purity and the dilution level with the product. I'll discuss this further within the text, however it is possible to create a negative reaction to your skin if not being cautious. But, with the correct product and the proper application, you can ease muscles tension, aches or even severe pain, when you apply it correctly.

Another method of using aromatherapy using essential oils can be to be able to enjoy the aroma of essential oils. Many people utilize droplets of essential oils on their pillows to get more restful nights or place them on tissue to breathe in the scent to clean their nasal passages. This can aid in avoiding allergies, and even to strengthen their lung capacity when trying to recover from pneumonia or have a bad case of flu.

Inhaling essential oils is an excellent way to get your mind off of things when experiencing headaches, mental issues or anxiety. The relaxing, soothing effect of the essential oil will allow you to breathe deeply into your body, and you'll feel calm and relaxed, as well as receiving the relief you've been searching for. Check to make sure that you've no allergy to essential oils are being used, as you don't want harm to yourself or trigger an adverse reaction.

Essential oils are utilized to aid in the treatment of any issue you may be confronting naturally. Naturally, it's not possible to repair bones by using essential oils, and you're certainly not going to treat cancer, but signs are able to be reduced and be removed in order to increase the possibilities of dealing with your issues naturally.

Don't want to be sucked into many medication and pills for ailments that can be solved at home with just five drops the essential oil. It's all about maintaining your body the most healthy possible, most natural manner feasible. Don't harm yourself by taking dangerous medications.

If you could find an organic and natural method to ease your soreness and pains, without medication, wouldn't that be the most effective way to go? You're not likely to experience exactly the same reaction from the medications you'll receive from essential oils, you'll taking the natural and healthy path. You don't have to be concerned about the negative effects of reactions or harm the medication could cause your body. It's a natural choice that you'll enjoy taking.

Chapter 12: Shopping for and Storing Essential oils

Purchase Essential Oils of Good Quality:

Pure, unadulterated essential oils can provide the highest in therapeutic benefits. Oils that were treated improperly, such as distilling from poor-quality crops, old, or adulterated oils could produce harmful side effects, or provide only a little therapeutic value. Be wary of claims that essential oils can be used for therapeutic or aromatherapy-grade since there is no government entity which regulates essential oils.

A few words to be aware of are natural identical oil, fragrance oil, as well as perfume oil. There are many vendors selling fragrance oils comprised of chemicals as well as essential oils, or all chemicals.

The best oils are usually sold in bottles of 4oz or less with dark-colored glass bottles. Be cautious about essential oils contained in clear glass bottles or plastic bottles. essential oils should be stored inside dark bottles of glass. The oils could cause plastic bottles to break down and cause contamination. Aluminum bottles with lining are okay, but do not purchase essential oils in bottles with an eyedropper made of rubber at the top, as essential oils could dissolve the plastic and cause it to become infected.

Find vendors who are offering the essential oils in samples to test before purchasing. If they're giving you many details about the essential oils your heart desires,, this will help to increase your confidence in the vendor.

Make an outline of any concerns or questions you might have, and send the vendors and see which ones provide you with the most comprehensive responses to your queries. This will assist you in the selection of a trustworthy online vendor.

Beware of sellers who are offering their essential oil at the same cost. This could be an indication that they're not high quality. Most essential oils are sold at diverse prices like citrus essential oils are generally lower than jasmine Rose and Neroli for example.

Check to observe that essential oils don't contain dust. This could indicate that they've been sitting for a lengthy period of time. Some oils lose their healing properties with time. Check you have the bottle sealed to ensure that they aren't damaged by other purchasers. Also ensure that the seller provides some samples for the oil essentials he's selling.

Do not purchase from sites or catalogs that don't mention specific botanical terms, the country that it is from, as well as the the method of extraction. A reputable aromatherapy supplier will have this information available.

Be cautious when purchasing items like essential oils purchased from sellers selling their products at carnivals festival, festivals, craft fairs or any other short-term events as these vendors will close and go onto the next event and leave customers with an item that they don't like and no place to return it.

The most effective method for introducing yourself into the aromatherapy world is to locate an established vendor. Start with a small amount of product. Once you've established that you're happy with the vendor, then you can increase the amount you order. Let your life become filled with delicious scents of the numerous essential oils for healing which are waiting to be tried!

Chapter 13: Essential Oils For Cleansing, Moisturizing & Toning

It is essential to use cleanser and toners on an everyday basis to keep your skin looking fresh and retain its original freshness and glow. There are a variety of cleanser on the market. Cleansers and toners may give you radiant and glowing skin, but the results is only short-lived. Additionally, they will harm the skin's internal structure. If you pick the wrong product, you may be a victim of a negative effect.

If you're searching for a scent-free and non-toxic cleanser, an oil blend is a great choice. They're cost-effective and give a long-lasting effect. The mixtures will get rid of the dirt that has been trapped and clean the skin as well as soothe the area that is inflamed. Essential oil cleanser will fulfill all the essential functions of a cleanser, but with extra advantages.

Certain essential oils such as lavender oil, bergamot oil, grapefruit oils and geranium oil possess powerful antiseptic properties that help your skin heal on the inside. If you're looking for anti-inflammatory properties, you should think about something like the chamomile oil or yarrow oil. For normal skin care you can choose from a range of alternatives, including frankincense oil the oil of sandalwood patchouli oil, benzoin oil, rose oil along with rosewood oil. These essential oils are beneficial for all types of skin.

These essential oils are great for toning your skin. To treat oily skin, apply lemongrass oil, lemon oil, rosemary oil along with peppermint oils. These essential oils you can mix them with water of flowers to reap the best benefits. You could think about anything that resembles the orange blossom or rose water. It is essential to create an appropriate blend to reap the advantages.

Recipes for essential oils blends for cleansing and toner

1. Citrus Cleanser

This cleanser from citrus is suitable for all skin types. It can help remove oily patches or dry, skin. For this blend, you'll need four drops of grapefruit oils, two drops of Geranium Oil 50g of cleanser, as well as three drops of essential oil of cedarwood.

2. Get your cleanser in shape

Cleansers that are a little cheery will help improve blood circulation and texture of the skin. It also helps in improving the skin's color. To make this mix, you'll require 4 drops of rosewood oil 3 drops palmarosa oils, 3 drops of grapefruit oils along with 50 grams of cleanser.

3. Forest toner

Forest Toner It is a relaxing blend that soothes and cools your skin. It's extremely beneficial in reducing the infection and inflammation associated with acne. To make this mix, you'll require 7 drops of the bergamot oil 5 drops sandalwood oil, 40ml rose water, and three drops of lavender oil.

Moisturizer

It is crucial to moisturize for radiant, youthful, and flawless skin into old age. Without moisturizers, you will not be able to keep your skin in the best way. A moisturizer can improve the appearance of your skin and reduce wrinkles and fine lines. It can slow the signs of ageing. If you're looking for an organic, fragrance-free and lanolin-free moisturizer you could try essential oils. Essential oils are extremely effective as moisturizers.

Essential oil blend recipes for moisturizing

1. Orange tree

The orange tree is a moisturizer that is beneficial to treat dry and flaky skin. If you suffer from dry skin and struggle to keep it in the balance, then you should think about using this moisturizer. To make this moisturizer, you'll need four drops orange oil, 10 drops sandalwood oil four drops of the neroli oil and 50g of moisturizer.

2. After-sun

A post-sun moisturizer can be very effective in treating sunburns. You can apply it to treat sunburns as a sunscreen lotion. It is also beneficial to treat dry, uncomfortable, and scaly patches of eczema. To make this cream, you'll require four drops of oil from yarrow, four drops of oil from cedarwood, eight drops lavender oil three drops of Bergamot oil and fifty grams of moisturizer.

3. Sunscreen lotion

You could also make your sunscreen lotion using essential oils. This mix can be more effective than the expensive sunscreen because it shields your skin from harmful ultraviolet rays from the sun. To make this natural sunscreen lotion, you'll require 1/2 cup olive oil and 1/4 cup coconut oil and 2 tablespoons of shea butter, 1 cup of beeswax pastilles one teaspoon of vitamin E oil tablespoons zinc oxide eight drops lavender oil five drops of helichrysum oils, and Geranium essential oil. All you need is to place all the ingredients above in the double boiler pan, excluding Zinc oxide. Reduce the heat until the ingredients melt. After that, you can take it from the flame and let it cool slightly and then add zinc oxide, mixing thoroughly. You can store the home-made sunscreen cream in a jar for later usage.

Chapter 14: Essential Oils Recipes For Mental Health

Mental health is just as vital as our physical health, if not more. This is because our brains are working all day long and it is the thing that holds us all together. If we overload it or put it under excessive stress, it is likely to be lost in our thoughts and nobody would want this. Essential oils have been proven to boost your mental well-being. If you're looking for an improved, faster and more clear brain, Essential oils could be the best way to take. If you can open your eyes to the idea, you'll be amazed by the ability to feel the benefits quickly. Five essential oils that can improve your mental clarity.

Rosemary

Juniper Berry

Sage Clary Sage Clary Sage

Basil

Peppermint

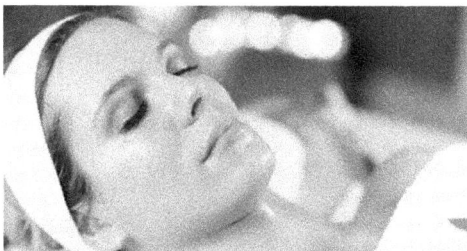

There are many ways of making use of essential oils to clear your mind. One of the most efficient methods to do this is to drop essential oils in an insulated pot filled with water. Then, you can warm the water until it's steaming and then turn off the temperature. You can put the pot back on the stove so that the oils disperse into the air and give your home the scents from the oils. If you are having difficult sleeping at night and don't want to awake the entire family by filling the home with essential oils, then you could try the candle diffuser. It's as simple as placing essential oils in the top of the bowl and then setting a tea light beneath it.

The tea light gives the sensation of heat that causes essential oils disperse into the air. Then, you'll be able to capture those incredible aromas that will help soothe you to sleep.

Rosemary Mist

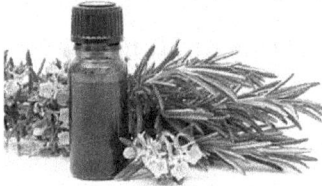

This can stimulate your senses , and is ideal after showering, but before drying off. It is best to apply it while your skin is still damp.

Ingredients

6 drops of rosemary essential oil

Spray bottle.

1 teaspoon olive oil.

5 ounces of water distilled.

1 sprig fresh rosemary

Procedure

Put all the ingredients in the spray bottle, shake it thoroughly to allow the ingredients to mix well.

You can spritz it as you'd like.

Massage oil for alertness

This oil massage will assist to boost your mental health and improve the alertness of your brain.

Ingredients

6 drops of ginger.

4 drops of Juniper Berry

5 drops of Grapefruit.

15ml of your favorite carrier oil.

Procedure

Blend all ingredients.

Make a few drops of it and massage the neck's back and around your temples, since it's all set to go.

Mental Clarity spray

The ability to focus is an essential aspect of good mental health, and that is the goal the spray is designed to attain.

Ingredients

50 drops of lemongrass.

20 drops of Cedarwood

40 drops of Niaouli.

40 drops of rosemary.

4 ounces of water, which is equivalent to 120 milliliters from pure water.

Procedure

Mix all essential oils, and after that, add the water.

Shake well.

The sprayer is and ready to use at any time you require it.

Spray of alertness

If you apply this spray and you'll be more alert and able to focus on what you're doing.

Ingredients

Forty Drops of Bergamot

25 drops of Lavender

40 drops of Grapefruit

30 drops of Juniper Berry

Forty Drops of Peppermint

4 8 ounces of pure water

Procedure

135

Blend all ingredients in a mist sprayer

Shake well.

Spray it with it using the sprayer that sprays mist.

Spray for refreshing

Our bodies and our minds must be refreshed every now and again in order to be ready to assume more responsibility.

Ingredients

4 oz. of water distilled

10 drops from Orange essential oil

5ml of essential oil Emulsifier

50 drops of essential lime oil

50 drops of Grapefruit essential oil

Procedure

Mix the emulsifier with all essential oils in the clean bottle.

Pour distilled water into the bottle.

Shake the bottle thoroughly.

The contents are spritzed in the air.

Always shake the bottle prior to you spray the contents. It is possible to use these ingredients in any diffuser, as long as you don't mess from the water and emulsifier. It is possible to use an amber bottle mix it and shake it thoroughly before putting a few drops into your diffuser.

Blending various essential oils you have at your disposal to serve different purposes is great as you control the ingredients you choose to use. Don't be discouraged for not having the time or energy to create these blends yourself. You can always purchase the products. Simply ask for the essential oils or blends of essential oils that you require. In any case, you will profit from these essential oils.

Chapter 15: Understanding The Proper Tools For Foraging

As with any venture having the appropriate tools and methods will increase your odds of success. When it comes to foraging, aside from knowing and utilizing your senses, a well-stocked toolkit can help you in choosing not only the most suitable herbs, but also the most effective ones as well. For you to begin this list of the tools you'll should prepare when foraging.

Tools for Picking

Even though your hands may be enough to harvest plants and herbs but it's still an excellent idea to employ the appropriate tool to pick, particularly when you're harvesting a herb that could be a cause of injury. Gardening gloves will help reduce irritation and protect you if you plan to pick your plants with your hands. Plastic mitts are also an excellent idea, especially in the case of a delicate plant.

For plants that must be cut from the lower part of the stem, and you don't wish to spend too much time taking the necessary section off, an excellent pair of scissors could assist. If you're trying to reach a higher point using a longer stick can significantly extend your reach. If you're searching for root matter, a smaller stick , or even a trowel will make the job much easier rather than working with your hands. For larger areas you may want to keep an extra shovel in your car in the event of.

Knives

Shears and knives are essential tools when hunting. Apart from harvesting, they are useful in cutting vines and branches that block your way. It is also useful as a tool for grasping as well as to mark your path through the forest.

Storage Containers

Another thing to plan ahead is your transportation containers. There may not be any specific containers in the case of hunting. In most cases, you will only require some containers that are covered and large poly bags for shopping, or freezer bags can suffice.

First Aid Kits

Since you're in the wild , and accidents can happen at any time It's best to be prepared should something happens while hunting. In preparing your first-aid kit, you could include the following items:

Tweezers, needles, and even tweezers are vital first aid tools for splinters and thorns.

Antiseptic products are useful when you're out foraging. Although bruises and slips are commonplace when out in the wild, carrying an antiseptic product, even if it's alcohol or povidone Iodine may aid in preventing infection.

Maintain a set of fresh plantain leaves in your initial aid kit. It will help you deal with insect bites and poison Ivy itchy rashes.

Rags and water

Being outside in the sun for a particular duration of time could cause your body to experience a some degree of dehydration. If you're planning to hunt be sure to take several bottles of water along for hydration. It's also important to wash your hands and tools. A rag or two can aid in cleaning up plants, berries or even the fingers of yours.

Illustrated Books

It is said that bringing handful of illustrated books is important to help you identify the correct plants and herbs. It's not essential to bring all of the books you'll need while you walk since they are able to carry some weight. Instead, you could carry one and put the rest in your car for a simpler cross-checking after you've gathered all the herbs needed.

Sun Protection

Exposure to the sun isn't healthy nor isn't safe. But, since foraging can make exposure to sun inevitable, it's recommended that you bring an appropriate hat or sunscreen. It's possible to apply the product, especially in the event that you'll spend several hours exploring the forest without under the trees' shade. Apart from sunscreen, you may need to carry a bag of spray for bugs to keep bugs away.

Magnifying Glass

There is no need for it, but having magnifying glasses with you when foraging trip to ensure you find the correct herbs. The magnifying glass allows you to examine small plants and herbs for identifiable characteristics that may make them stand out from other members of their family and species. The difference in hair color or tiny holes in the stem could be all that you need to recognize the herb. Since your eyes can be limited what they can see an excellent magnifying glass will help make the task simpler.

Proper clothing

There aren't any specific guidelines for what you can and should not wear while hunting but the goal is to wear something that's safe and comfortable. Clothing with lengthy sleeves and pants that are long are a good choice as they will help keep insects from biting your skin and the thorny plants aren't damaging your skin. It's also beneficial to wear a scarf to give you extra protection from the sun. If you're on your feet, you stick to footwear and socks.

Snacks

It's not necessary to carry lots of food, especially in the event that you'll spend most of your time looking for plants and herbs. However, as the task is often tedious and tiring It is recommended to carry snacks to munch on as you hunt.

Candies and biscuits are a great way to prevent the occurrence of hypoglycemia, or low blood sugar that typically occurs when you perform excessive physical activities. Since the effects caused by hypoglycemia, especially when not corrected immediately, could be fatal, it is important to be proactive in preventing it from occurring at all.

Chapter 16: The Essential Oils and their uses

This chapter will list various essential oils commonly utilized and the purposes they are utilized to serve. Each essential oil has its own characteristic or another that will benefit us in some manner. Understanding these properties will allow you to gain knowledge and use aromatherapy to reap the maximum benefits. After you have gone through this process, you'll be amazed at how beneficial essential oils can be.

Peppermint - This essential oil provides a refreshing and stimulating effects. It can be used to alleviate problems such as nausea and bad breath due to its aroma. Inflammation of the stomach or PMS symptoms could be treated by using this oil. The essential oil peppermint is believed to aid in the treatment of headaches and colds. It also helps with the ability to concentrate.

CloveEssential oil is thought to be among the top choices of dentists. It helps with problems like bad breath and offers relief from pain in the mouth or gums. It is a common ingredient in balms, and it soothes nasal congestions and headaches. Clove oil is also beneficial in treating digestive issues and is applied to bug bites or scrapes.

Lavender - This essential oil is also very well-known due to its attractive scent and health benefits. Acne sunburn, acne, etc. can be treated using this oil because it is a potent blend of antibacterial properties. It also does wonders for hair, making it stronger and healthier after regular massages.

Rosemary The most well-known essential oil comes with numerous benefits. It's extremely effective in treating digestive issues like constipation or cramps as well as indigestion. It acts as a disinfectant and also anti-microbial. It is employed to maintain oral hygiene and as skin care products for toning as well as dry and flaky skin. It is beneficial for hair care because it encourages hair growth and treating scalp flaky with hair dandruff. The oil is also thought to boost mood and increase mental energy.

Tea Tree -This vital oil is extremely effective in treating infections caused by bacteria both externally and internally. It aids in healing wounds more quickly and increases the immune system. It can help with measles, colds and other viral infections that could affect the body. Hair health is also improved by this oil because hair loss and dandruff is decreased. The oil's essential properties have positive effects on hormonal balance, as well.

Lemon - One of the most commonly utilized vital oils that is used in the kitchen is lemon. It's used for treating problems with the skin, such as acne and oily skin. It also improves the complexion but it should not be used just prior to going under the sun. It is relaxing and refreshing.

It helps in relieving discomfort and reducing inflammation throughout the body.

NeroliEssential oil has a positive effect and can help to manage signs of depression. The application of the oil helps to reduce the appearance of scars and marks. It can also be employed to treat gastritis-related symptoms.

EucalyptusEssential oil is a potent blend of properties that range between anti-inflammatory and antibacterial. The antiseptic effect makes it ideal for the healing of burns, cuts as well as sores. It can also be used to treat ailments that affect respiratory systems like sinusitis, colds and asthma and so on. It functions as a stimulant, and it improves the mood and relieves stress-related symptoms.

PineThe essential oil Pine is another favorite of aromatherapists. It is antibacterial and has antiseptic properties that help solve issues like acne and eczema aswell being able to kill other bacteria. The oil also has an analgesic property that improves metabolism. Joint pain can be relieved with this.

Rose- The aroma released by this essential oil has been a favorite option. It is an energy booster and is particularly popular with women. The oil can help to get rid of mood swings and is believed to help improve hormonal imbalances. It also provides relief of PMS symptoms.

Sesame- Sesame essential oil is quite beneficial for skin problems. It's very moisturizing and is very effective on dry skin and gives it the healthy look. The oil helps to keep skin moisturized and also shields against harmful UV rays thanks because of its SPF.

Sandalwood- This essential oil can provide the ability to relax and cool effect. It aids in relaxing the mind and ease insomnia or anxiety. Its astringent properties make it suitable for the skin. It can be found in creams and lotions in the form of an additive. It is particularly beneficial for sensitive and dry type of skin.

Calendula- Even though the scent isn't very well-known however, this essential oil has numerous beneficial properties. It can be used to treat skin conditions like acne and is suitable for those with sensitive skin. It can also help to tone the skin and is beneficial for Psoriasis.

GrapefruitEssential oil that is both energizing and cleansing. It is a powerful antidepressant that has an elevating impact. The antioxidant component makes it a good choice for strengthening the immune system, and helps fight against diseases such as premature aging, tissue degeneration and so on. It also has antimicrobial properties that is useful for a variety of uses. It is used on injuries and cuts because of its antiseptic properties.

Clary sage - It has antibacterial properties that help combat infections within the digestive tract, excretory system as well as other organs. As an antidepressant, this oil eases stress and anxiety. It is also utilized to treat spasms, and soothes nerves.

The Ylang ylang oil isn't widely acknowledged, yet it has a lot of benefits. It assists in relaxing the mind and body and reduces mood swings. It also aids in maintaining healthy skin and is utilized to treat skin irritations as well as inflammations. It also treats wounds and stops infections and speeds the process of healing. It is believed to have a positive effect on decreasing blood pressure, and beneficial for the nervous system, too.

Geranium Essential oil anti-bacterial and astringent characteristics. It is effective in addressing skin issues if they are sensitive to acne and oily. It also decreases the appearance of scars and marks and helps reduce bloating, inflammation and redness. It is also believed to fight aging because it affects the blood vessels, in a manner which reduces wrinkles that appear on the skin. The symptoms of PMS can also be alleviated with the use in the form of oil from Geranium.

AngelicaThe essential oil utilized to treat spasms that are that are caused by various illnesses. It is also useful in dealing with stomach pains and gastritis. It's great for regular sweating and urination. It also aids in purifying the blood. The harmful substances and toxins are eliminated through the system. It is also beneficial for helping menstrual cycle normalization and helps relieve PMS symptoms. It also acts as a diuretic as well as a beneficial digestive oil.

Wintergreen This essential oil can help reduce pain and soothes the body. It's great for relieving signs of tension and stress. It also helps reduce the frequency and severity of spasms. It also functions as a diuretic agent and aids in cleansing the body of toxic substances. It also acts as an astringent that helps smooth the skin.

Fir needle - This essential oil is antiseptic, and is utilized to treat infections and increasing the body's immune. It also assists the body flush out harmful toxins and cleanses. The oil acts as a pain relief. Its pleasant aroma is what makes it so popular, and makes you feel fresh and buoyed. It's also useful to ease congestion.

ThymeEssential oil commonly employed in soaps, perfumes and other products. It provides an energizing cleanse to our body. It is an antispasmodic particularly in muscle cramps. It also helps with conditions like arthritis or rheumatism. It can also be used to treat wounds and also as an anti-bacterial. It assists in flushing out toxic substances in the body.

Mullein Essential oil that numbs the nerves and offers relief from headaches, toothaches and headaches. It also helps reduce inflammation that can be present in the digestive system. It also defend against infections and is also a disinfectant. It also provides relief from asthmatic, cough, congestion symptoms, etc. The oil can ease the tension in muscles and nerves and reduce blood pressure.

Myrrhh- This essential oil is antimicrobial as well being antiviral. It aids in fighting colds Pox, poisoning and other diseases. It also helps fight fungal infections that can affect the body. The oil can also help in sweating to eliminate toxic substances that build up in the body. The oil is able to ease gas, which causes the stomach pain and causes digestive issues. It also improves your immunity.

You can clearly see, there are many essential oils, and they all have numerous beneficial properties. In this article, we will discuss essential oils that work best for specific purposes, as shown below.

Hair growth oils

lavender essential oil

lemon essential oil

geranium essential oil

essential oil of rosemary

Oils for disinfection

Essential oil of thyme

Essential oil of tea tree

oregano essential oil

Melrose essential oil

Oils to heal wounds

Lavender essential oil

Tea tree essential oil

Melrose essential oil

Oils for treating itching

Peppermint essential oil

Lavender essential oil

The use of oils to prevent bleeding

Geranium essential oil

Oils to treat acne

Eucalyptus essential oil

Geranium essential oil

Melaleuca essential oil

Oils to fight aging

Sandalwood essential oil

Lavender essential oil

Frankincense essential oil

Rose essential oil

Oils for digestion

Peppermint essential oil

Fennel essential oil

Coriander essential oil

Ginger essential oil

Metabolic oils

Grapefruit essential oil

Lemon essential oil

Peppermint essential oil

Ginger essential oil

Oils for PMS

Ylang ylang essential oil

Cedarwood essential oil

Fennel essential oil

Chamomile essential oil

Clary essential oil of sage

Lavender essential oil

The oils are a great way to relax muscles

Basil essential oil

Lavender essential oil

Peppermint essential oil

Cypress essential oil

Grapefruit essential oil

Oils to treat skin

Neroli essential oil

Ylang ylang essential oil

Myrrh essential oil

Lavender essential oil

Frankincense essential oil

Lemon essential oil

The oil for fever

Eucalyptus essential oil

Lavender essential oil

Tea tree essential oil

Peppermint essential oil

Rosemary essential oil

Oils for heartburn

Eucalyptus essential oil

Fennel essential oil

Peppermint essential oil

Oils to boost protection

Tea tree essential oil

Lemon essential oil

Chamomile essential oil

Lavender essential oil

Oils for sun protection

Essential oil of almond

Carrot seed essential oil

Oils to treat cough

Eucalyptus essential oil

Thyme essential oil

Oils to treat constipation

Rosemary essential oil

Lemon essential oil

Peppermint essential oil

Oils for insomnia

Lavender essential oil

Clary essential oil of sage

Sandalwood essential oil

Chapter 17: A History Behind Aromatherapy. Background Behind Aromatherapy

Aromatic substances have been used for many years to serve a variety of purposes, including rituals of worship and medicinal use. Of course, during the past, they didn't have access to the steam-distilled products we have in the present. Because steam distillation wasn't invented until the Biblical time, the use of aromatic materials actually started in the 11th century, when the scientist Ibn Sina discovered steam distillation. It is believed that steam distillation was utilized in King Tut's time, which was around 2300 years back. If it had been employed in the past it would have been an unrefined solvent that had the lowest yield and not even close to the ones we can access in the present. The advancement of technology and the knowledge we have gained has brought us closer to making better products that can deliver positive results.

What would you think if I said the essential oils were in use for centuries? Yes, its true and works. Aromatherapy is a segment of this tree as it is a centuries-old practice. it uses essential oils from plants (Essential oil) to promote overall health and wellbeing. It is part of an "holistic therapeutic scale" makes use of natural ingredients such as clay, herbs, mud Jojoba, and even vegetable oil.

There are also Aromatherapists in your area. They aren't exorcists or shamans who can magically heal your body, but they will revive you. Have you heard about massages that are aromatherapy? Oil is applied on the skin and, when applied by a professional the muscles will be relaxed. Essential oils can also be used to improve the quality of air. It is common to find spas are equipped with automated sprays or diffusers within their facilities.

Certain aromatherapists claim that essential oils have the capacity to stimulate nerve receptors inside the nostrils. The stimulation helps relax the brain because endorphins are released as well as they provide the feeling of satisfaction and peace. When a person inhale the scent from essential oils, nerves that line their nose send electrical signals to the region of the brain that regulates emotions and memory. The stimulation produces the relaxing feeling that many people experience.

What Essential Oils are Beneficial for?

There are now a myriad of misconceptions about essential oils and aromatherapy. Essential oils constitute the primary ingredient in aromatherapy . They are liquids that are concentrated, and are extracted naturally from the roots, bark fruit and flowers. Each essential oil are unique in their properties and features a distinctive smell. These various types of essential oils are used for different purposes; Here are the various types of essential oils and their most commonly used ones:

* Eucalyptus is used in the preparation of topical products, this oil is pure and revitalizing oil.

* Ginger: It is known for its ability to reduce headaches and can also boost your appetite.

*Juniper Berry The berry of the Juniper tree is thought to help strengthen and restore the immune system.

* Lavender: The oil is utilized in a variety of ways including baths, lotions and even baths and it has a distinct scent that people enjoy.

* Lemon Cheerful is the perfect term to define this essential oil. It is uplifting and refreshing. Some prefer to dilute the oil before applying it on the skin.

*Peppermint: a stimulating scent that can rejuvenate your body and help keep cool.

*Rosemary: Often used in households It is used in shampoos and soaps.

Sage is a very strong scent. A couple of drops is usually enough.

*Spearmint: Essential oil that is refreshing and cool that can open your tight pores when you include this oil in warm bath.

*Tea Tree Oil: Tea tree oil is able to be used to treat fungi, bacteria viruses, and boost the immune system.

How to Apply Essential Oils to treat hair and Skin Care

The Body Spray can mix 3-8 essential oils into a bottle along with some water. If you're using a citrus-based product, make sure you don't use it without dilution heavily the oil by adding water. The oils of citrus are sensitive to light and can leave your skin prone to sunburn. It is possible to use lemon oil as well as orange oils. Orange oil, on the other hand is much more potent and refreshing . However, the oil you choose to use is dependent on your preferences.

Shampoo: Do have that itchy scalp? Try just a few drops of the cedarwood or on basil to your shampoo. Cedarwood, lavender, and basil are wonderful to soothe a dry scalp. Additionally, basil can do miracles to increase your hair's volume.

Skin cream It doesn't matter what skin cream you're using, regardless of whether it's regular or anti-aging, you can mix in 1-2 drops of rose. Rose oil can make your skin appear radiant and offer great support used in conjunction with the cream you are using.

You could even prepare your own oils. If you're making use of almonds, apricots sesame, jojoba kernel, apricot as well as wheat germ oil you'll need to add about two drops of each essential oil. It will add the health benefits of the oil and you'll be awed by the aroma.

What should you not add to your bath water? Use as little as 6 drops of essential oils in your bath, but stay clear of the culinary oils such as peppermint, lemongrass, and cinnamon because they may cause irritations on the skin.

Which essential oil can help your hair grow?

Lavender is not just a pleasant scent but is also loved by many. It is a popular choice of Aromatherapists. Lavender has been proven to boost hair growth when used frequently. Massage your scalp using lavender 3 times per week and you'll see the improvement. The hair will begin to grow thickerand more dense, and you'll be able to observe that your scalp is no longer itching if you suffer from itchy scalp.

Here's an amazing recipe for hair:

1. A half-cup of olive oil (not too hot)

2. Mix in around 10 drops (or depending on your preference) of lavender oil. Blend in approximately 10 drops (or as you like).

3. Apply the mixture on your hair and gently massage your scalp.

4. Wrap a hot towel over your head, relax and unwind for around 20 minutes.

5. Make sure to follow it up with a natural , natural shampoo and conditioner

Essential oils you must have to stay clear of

Many believe it is because the pain caused by essential oils on the skin is merely skin detoxing, but this is not the case. If you experience an itch on your skin that is not the body detoxing it is your body telling you "What is going on? Let it go". The rash can be a sign to your body's message that this oil isn't beneficial therefore, don't classify an itchy rash as an indication of detox.

There are numerous essential oils, each special and beneficial, however not all of them are able to use on the face as certain oils may cause skin irritations or allergies.

Here's a list essential oils you should avoid applying on your skin:

1. Bitter Almond

2. Calamus

3. Horseradish

4. Mugwort

5. Mustard

6. Rue

7. Yellow Camphor

8. Savin

9. Southernwood

10. Tansy

Where to Purchase Essential Oils and Aromatherapy

This book is an introduction to a vast field of essential oils and aromatherapy. I hope you enjoy this book!

If you enjoyed the book, I'd would appreciate it if the book had me a review. You can do this by clicking here I'm sure you'd like to write an online review.

You can purchase essential oils at any time, but you must be aware since not all sellers are selling high quality products. A lot of people extract oils by themselves but in today's world this method might not be the best choice for you. It is possible to search the web to find the best manufacturer, and in case you don't find one, you could always visit one of the stores that provides essential oils.

Chapter 18: The Buyer's Guide

To become an informed consumer and buy top quality essential oils to use in aromatherapy, you must know what makes the best quality essential oil from one of poor quality and how to pick a trustworthy vendor to acquire the finest products. These tips can help you gain maximum worth.

Get the best quality products at the lowest price.

Although numerous stores sell essential oils in stores and online however, the quality of these oils may differ. It's tempting to buy essential oils from companies which offer them at the most affordable price. It is the quality and purity of oil that are crucial for the best therapeutic results Do not purchase the cheapest , but ensure the highest quality. The price alone isn't a guarantee of high-quality, but it could be. Professionally-trained vendors who spend endless hours searching for quality oils, and pay expensive costs to test their oils and give free samples upon request , should be offering higher prices for their oils than those who sell oils they've obtained from the most affordable sources. Always opt for pure, natural oils that originate by sustainable, fresh sources and distributed by reliable dealers.

Pure essential oils are preferred over mix

There are a variety of essential oil mixtures for purchase. These mix an assortment of oils to treat a variety of illnesses. Since the structure and chemical composition of essential oils are very delicate and complex, premixed solutions aren't always the most efficient. Be sure to look for "100 100% essential oil" on the label. Beware of terms like "fragrance oil,"" "nature similar oil" as well as "perfume oil." These terms indicate that the product you are looking at is not a pure one essential oil. Purchase pure oils in single bottles and mix them by yourself. Do not use essential oils dilute by vegetable oils. To test this, put some drops of essential oil over a small piece paper. If the oil creates an oily stain, it's probably been dilute with vegetable oil.

Purchase only a small amount

In addition to the financial implications, there are two main reasons you should purchase only small amounts of essential oils.

Just a tiny amount just a few drops of oil essential is required at any given moment.

Essential oils diminish their potency quickly . They also are able to be used for a limited time Buy fresh and use it quickly.

Test before purchasing even if it's an unpaid trial

Find vendors who are providing samples you can test before purchasing. Request additional samples (don't demand an entire sample and honestly request at least 2-4 oils you're genuinely looking to purchase). The aim is to find out whether this is a seller that you feel comfortable with without having to pay for huge orders that you may not be satisfied with. Look for vendors that provide comprehensive details on every oil they sell, more so if they can educate you on the methods of extraction of these oils. Since it's expensive and time-consuming for the vendors to offer samples, and certain vendors get a large amount of inquiries for samples at no cost, they have to charge a minimal fee to provide samples. This does not reflect badly on the seller.

Keep it in a safe place

Purchase high-quality oils in sizes of 4 1 oz. or smaller in dark colored glass. Make sure to store the oils you make yourself in an area that is cool and dark because the direct heat and sunlight can ruin the delicate chemical properties. Certain vendors also offer more oils in bottles made of aluminum. Aluminum is thought to be safe in the event that the interior container is lined. Beware of buying essential oils with an eyedropper made of rubber in the top of the bottle because the oil may disintegrate the rubber dropper and be contaminated.

Be vigilant when you make purchases made online

When buying oils online, to ship large quantities of essential oils, specifically plastic containers to prevent breakage and cut down on shipping costs. Essential oils will dissolve plastic bottles which means that the potency of oil may decrease in quality faster. If you receive oils in clear glass or plastic make sure you move the oils into dark colored glass bottles therefore it's a smart idea to have empty bottles available. If you buy from a seller who is shipping in plastic ask them about the length of time the oil has been kept in plastic bottles prior to shipping. It is best to choose suppliers who transfer the oil to plastic right before shipping.

Don't be fooled by false promises

There isn't a governmental regulatory organization that certifies or grades essential oils to be "therapeutic Grade" as well as "aromatherapy quality." Beware of suppliers who promote their essential oils under the words "therapeutic grade" or "aromatherapy grade..

Chapter 19: The Difference Between Fragrance Oils and Essential Oils

The primary distinction of essential oils and fragrance oil lies in that they are both a nature substance and perfume oils are manufactured. Both have advantages and disadvantages.

Fragrance oils are more affordable to manufacture because they are synthetic however they don't have the benefits that essential oils can provide. Contrarily essential oils are costly to obtain in huge amounts but they do offer the benefits of volatile constituents, which cannot be replicated in a synthetic manner.

Fragrance oils, also known as perfume oils which are also called, are synthetic scents. They are created to mimic the smell of natural product such as coffee. Because of their low production cost, they are often used for the production of cosmetics, perfumes, and flavorings. Candle makers and soap makers, for instance always make use of fragrance oils. While essential oils can certainly be used in the production of these items, it's not going to make much sense as the fragrance oil is a more affordable alternative.

Essential oils are beneficial for health.

There are numerous benefits associated with the use of essential oils. Let's take a to look at some of these advantages.

Zero Side Effects

Because essential oils originate from plant parts they do not have any adverse negative effects associated with the use of essential oils. This is why it is that the majority of people choose to make use of aromatherapy instead of conventional therapies and pharmaceutical drugs due to the many adverse negative effects that result from the latter. Regular use of essential oils will enhance your well-being. It is only necessary to make sure that you don't suffer from any allergic reactions to essential oils.

Accessible and Cheap

It is always best to select essential oils instead of prescription drugs as they cost more than the first. Essential oils can be purchased from shelves at the grocery store that you frequent and are priced higher than what you might think. If they are stored correctly the oils will last at most five years. If you decide to switch to essential oils, you'll find that your expenses are reduced by a large amount from the amount they were at with pharmaceutical medications.

Market Access

Essential medications do not require to be purchased from the drug store because there is no need for prescriptions from your physician. They can be purchased at any local supermarket. If, however, you'd prefer to extract the oils yourself then you can follow the procedure described in the previous paragraph.

Chronic Illness

The majority of doctors prescribe pharmaceutical medications for patients suffering from chronic conditions like arthritis or sinusitis. It is essential to use these medications regularly to ease the pain you experience. To stay clear of the negative side negative effects of the medication you should consider switching to essential oils because they can have a lasting effect on your body.

You can apply the oils into your joints or around your temples to alleviate discomfort. Essential oils, also known as mixtures made of them, are utilized in place of prescription drugs to treat headaches, colds or other ailments. There are a few blends listed in the book to aid in getting rid of colds quickly.

Secure

Each drug prescribed by your physician includes a list of directions that need to be adhered to. To ensure the medication doesn't cause any adverse consequences.

Since essential oils don't cause any adverse consequences, you don't have any list of guidelines that must be adhered to. They can be used for bathing (bath bombs) in combination with other oils or even use them without anxiety.

Manage Anxiety and Stress

In the present, nearly everyone is stressed out about their lives or jobs and this leads to the creation of anxiety, and sometimes depression. The majority of people write depression and anxiety off as stress and then continue to work at the same time. This could have an adverse effect to their health. Doctors frequently prescribe antidepressants that can help people manage depression and anxiety However, these medications are also known to cause adverse consequences on the body. To avoid these problems it is recommended to utilize essential oils to bring your nerves. Essential oils are believed to provide a relaxing effect on the body, thereby relieving any stress you might be experiencing.

Conclusion

I am very happy to relay this knowledge to you. I am extremely happy to have learned and are able to implement these methods in the future.

I hope that this book was helpful in helping you understand the importance of essential oils and how they can help you with your natural beauty and health issues, without the risk.

It is now time to begin with this information and hopefully lead a healthy, completely natural lifestyle!

Do not be someone who reads the information and does not apply it. the methods included in this book will only be beneficial if you implement the strategies! If you know someone who might benefit from the advice that is provided, please inform them of the book.

Thanks and best of luck!

www.ingramcontent.com/pod-product-compliance
Lightning Source LLC
Chambersburg PA
CBHW060333030426
42336CB00011B/1320